Geriatric Orthopaedics

Geriatric Orthopaedics

edited by

MICHAEL DEVAS, M.Chir., F.R.C.S.

Royal East Sussex Hospital, Hastings, Sussex

1977

ACADEMIC PRESS

London   New York   San Francisco

A Subsidiary of Harcourt Brace Jovanovich, Publishers

ACADEMIC PRESS INC. (LONDON) LTD.
24/28 Oval Road
London NW1

United States Edition published by
ACADEMIC PRESS INC.
111 Fifth Avenue
New York, New York 10003

Library of Congress Catalog Card Number: 76-24427
ISBN: 0-12-213750-7

Contributors

C. G. Attenborough, M.Chir., F.R.C.S.,
Consultant Orthopaedic Surgeon,
Royal East Sussex Hospital and Hastings Health District.

Harold S. Brodribb, B.M., B.Ch., D.M.(Oxon), M.R.C.S., L.R.C.P.,
Honorary Consultant Physician
In charge of Hastings Diabetic Clinic 1945-75.

Michael Devas, M.Chir., F.R.C.S.,
Consultant Orthopaedic Surgeon,
Royal East Sussex Hospital and Hastings Health District.

Ann M. Haines, M.B., Ch.B., D.C.H., F.F.A.R.C.S.,
Consultant Anaesthetist,
Royal East Sussex Hospital and Hastings Health District.

M. R. P. Hall, M.A., B.M., F.R.C.P.(Lond.Edin.),
Professor of Geriatric Medicine,
University of Southampton,
Honorary Consultant Physician, Southampton Group of Hospitals.

R. I. Irvine, M.A., M.D., F.R.C.P.,
Consultant Physician,
St. Helens Hospital and Hastings Health District.

Harry Middleton, F.F.A.R.C.S.,
Consultant Anaesthetist,
Royal East Sussex Hospital and Hastings Health District.

T. Strouthidis, M.B., M.R.C.P.(London),
Consultant Physician,
St. Helens Hospital and Hastings Health District.

Ivan Williams, F.R.C.P., D.Phys.Med.,
Consultant Rheumatologist,
Tunbridge Wells Health District.

Editor's Foreword

The study of geriatric orthopaedics started at Hastings out of necessity. The south coast of Britain has a very dense geriatric population and Hastings was no exception. The orthopaedic unit was small and it was apparent that few patients would be admitted for elective surgery unless existing methods of rehabilitating the geriatric orthopaedic patient were improved to allow a much quicker discharge from hospital than was usual at that time.

This book is a description of the methods developed and used at Hastings in the treatment of geriatric orthopaedic patients. The methods appear to have overcome many of the problems of treating and rehabilitating elderly patients with fractures, or with other orthopaedic conditions, so that an early discharge from hospital has become the rule. The most important principle in the achievement of this is to have teamwork; without it there could have been no progress. By the co-operation of physicians, surgeons and anaesthetists it has been possible to maintain a brisk rate of admission and discharge; it has shown that the ability to work together has prevented the orthopaedic beds being blocked by elderly patients. The book describes also how certain new surgical techniques have improved the speed of rehabilitation and improved function. Always the goal has been to achieve a satisfactory quality of life for all old people and to return them to independence. There has been no attempt to rehabilitate too much, such as attempting to obtain full movements in the joints of old people when it is not needed: all that is necessary is a quick return to the activities of daily living, because this brings independence.

In the practice of geriatric orthopaedics one of the most important tenets is to keep the patient up. This means that any orthopaedic technique used on any old person must be so reliable that the patient can walk immediately after the operation; nevertheless these methods must also be simple.

Some of the methods of treatment have not been described before while others have, but there is nothing in this book that is theoretical or untried. It is a record of how the problems of the elderly are overcome, on a day to day basis, while they are in an orthopaedic ward.

Particular attention has been given to social problems because their solution is often the key to the door of rapid discharge.

Without teamwork this book could never have been written. It is a great tribute to the whole team—physiotherapists, occupational therapists, social workers, secretaries, and, above all, the nursing staff—because without their full co-operation and assistance the patient's path to recovery would have been tortuous and tedious.

My very sincere thanks go to Mrs. Audrey Caswell for her invaluable secretarial assistance with the preparation of the book and also I am most grateful to Mrs. Ellen Lilico for proof reading.

April 1977   M.D.

Introduction

M. R. P. HALL

Professor of Geriatric Medicine, University of Southampton.
Honorary Consultant Physician, Southampton Group of Hospitals

It is well known that the incidence of disease increases with age and several major conditions often coexist in a single individual. The management of illness in an old person is complex. Charcot in his lectures on Chronic and Senile Diseases, given almost 100 years ago, stressed that senile pathology would only be properly understood if it was studied as a special subject. The speciality of Geriatric Medicine was born in Britain a little over 40 years ago and, since the health service, has grown so that at the present time there is hardly a single health district without a specialist geriatric department. These are headed by one or more consultant physicians who have become expert in understanding senile pathology and managing the problems which result from it. These problems are diffuse, involving the health of the individual in its fullest sense; that of his physical, mental and social well being. Assessment of an individual's ability to function against his social and environmental background becomes a matter of prime importance.

Assessment is a word often used in geriatric medicine and one which is often misunderstood by doctors, nurses, and those members of the professions supplementary to medicine who are without the specialty. These colleagues relate the word more to the social and environmental aspects of care than to the clinical, whereas correctly used it means accurate clinical diagnosis of physical and mental disease; its treatment; rehabilitation of the patient to his best functional level; and then his resettlement in the community. If, as has already been said, several major conditions coexist in a single individual, several specialists may be involved in both diagnosis and treatment. Further, rehabilitation and resettlement will involve others, so that the whole management of the patient's illness will be a team exercise with many people contributing to the successful outcome.

Because clinical medicine is the base upon which the care of the elderly is founded, it is inevitable that geriatric medicine is a diffuse subject impinging on many different specialties. Patients will present with the disorders of internal medicine or of general surgery, psychiatry, urology, ophthalmology, or orthopaedics. In the practice of his discipline the physician in geriatric medicine will have to liaise and work closely with many colleagues who practice in different disciplines and who also have a considerable contribution to make to the management and treatment of the illnesses of old age and the health of the individual elderly person.

With increasing numbers of elderly in the population any health service must be comprehensive in the care it provides; and as numbers increase, so more and more doctors in disciplines other than geriatric medicine will become involved in the care of the elderly. It is estimated that the number of people over the age of 75 years in Britain will increase by almost one million during the next twenty years, while the number over 85 years will increase by a quarter of a million in the next thirty years. It is already well known that the greatest morbidity occurs in those over 75 years. Community surveys, for instance, suggest that the incidence of senile dementia in people over 85 years will be of the order of 25%. If all these were to be cared for in institutions then an additional 50 000—60 000 places would need to be provided. Obviously, therefore, the provision of a psychiatric service for the elderly is of great importance and in many places psychiatrists are developing a special interest in the elderly and are co-operating with physicians in geriatric medicine to plan and provide a special service.

With ageing, changes occur in other systems apart from the brain and, as a consequence, on the intellect. Some changes are physiological while others are pathological. Diminution of vision and hearing as well as a reduction in other aspects of sensory perception make the individual less aware of his environment. As a result he confines his activity and by doing less becomes less mobile. This tendency to immobility is accompanied by an increase in sway and an inability to correct movements once these have been initiated. To fall is therefore common and this will sometimes lead to injury, which in turn will need treatment.

Like most things, geriatric medicine began in a small way. Like most people, consultant physicians interested in the elderly concentrated on things that interested them. The service that resulted was often the work of an enthusiast who by his energy and ability to work with and stimulate others developed a model which could be copied and transposed to other areas. Hastings has for many years had a famous geriatric service which is visited by many people from all over the world. Part of the success of this service, and a model which should be copied much more widely, is the close co-operation that exists between orthopaedic surgeons and physicians in geriatric medicine. This has happened because both physician and surgeon realised their close co-operation would benefit the elderly patients. This book, long overdue, is the fruit of this union and clearly states the reasons why such liaison is necessary.

One of the prime health needs of any old person is for comfortable survival. Bone and joint disease is an uncomfortable state and the sooner the elderly patient can be made comfortable the better he will be. Because we recognise that the management of an elderly person is complex, one might have thought that the model geriatric orthopaedic unit described in Chapter

14 would have been a standard provision in every district general hospital. Most physicians and surgeons would agree that a close liaison between geriatric and orthopaedic departments must exist, yet this happens only in a few places. This may be because some orthopaedic surgeons think that a fracture of the upper femur, one of the commonest problems, is simply an incident in a complex socio-medical disease so that the role of the orthopaedic surgeon is minor to that of the physician in geriatric medicine.

Alternatively some physicians in geriatric medicine may feel that their role, once they have instructed the orthopaedic surgeon and his team on the proper management and rehabilitation of the elderly patient, is one of consultant in the difficult case. Orthopaedic surgeons and physicians in geriatric medicine are both busy groups with big work loads and both viewpoints can be defended. However friendly the arguments that cross disciplinary boundaries it is often the patient who is the loser. Further, as the authors of this book have clearly shown, the scope of orthopaedic surgery and geriatric medicine for the benefit of the elderly patient is immense. Much can be gained from a joint approach, not only to promote the comfortable survival of the patient in his own home, but also for research into his problems from many points of view.

Let us hope it will stimulate both orthopaedic surgeons and physicians in geriatric medicine to think again about the problems of their patients and, with their colleagues in rehabilitation medicine, consider how best they can achieve a joint approach, even if they do not actually copy the Hastings model, so that their patients, like Ulysees, may say:—

I am a part of all that I have met;
Yet all experience is an arch wherethro'
Gleams that untravell'd world, whose margin fades
For ever and for ever when I move.
How dull it is to pause, to make an end,
To rust unburnished, not to shine in use!
As tho' to breathe were life

Come, my friends,
'Tis not too late to seek a newer world.

Contents

Contents

1

Principles of Geriatric Orthopaedics

MICHAEL DEVAS

Geriatric orthopaedics is a combination of the principles of medicine and orthopaedics applied to the elderly. The surgeon alone cannot achieve the level of care necessary to rehabilitate the elderly, with their many concomitant illnesses, unless he brings in the skills of geriatric medicine and all its ancillary methods of after care and support.

The principles of either the medicine or the surgery used on the geriatric patient are the same as those at any other age, but it is the application of the principles that is different.

In the elderly existence on its own has many problems with which to contend: the addition of an illness or injury may cause the loss of the ability to continue to live an independent life. Geriatric orthopaedics can only be successful by taking into account the problems that beset the elderly patient and by overcoming each difficulty with the least delay possible. Only then will the geriatric orthopaedic patient have the best chance of returning home to continue to enjoy an independent existence with a satisfactory quality of life.

The orthopaedic surgeon can only organise the orthopaedic care necessary for his ill and debilitated patients, and because the geriatric physician has far greater facilities for medical rehabilitation and after-care than is found in an orthopaedic unit it is logical to combine the two disciplines.

Speed is absolutely essential because the longer the elderly remain in hospital the more difficult is their ultimate discharge to the same level of activity and independence as before. This aspect of treatment is well recognised by the geriatrician.

Because there is a very large elderly population undiluted by younger generations in the Hastings district it is necessary to maintain the rapid progress of geriatric orthopaedic patients through the acute wards by applying the principles of orthopaedic surgery and geriatric medicine with the utmost vigour. This prevents the stagnation of geriatric patients in

1

hospital because of failure in rehabilitation. Most important of all is the close liaison of both specialities, and, at Hastings, this has resulted in a geriatric orthopaedic unit which has been found indispensable for the rehabilitation of the ill, elderly and decrepit patients, particularly after emergency orthopaedic surgery. The unit is described later in this book in Chapter 14.

By studying geriatric methods it became very obvious that the elderly are better treated by being up than by being in bed. This means that the orthopaedic surgeon must deal with any lesion in such a way that the patient can be got up forthwith. To use the most common problem as an example, all old people with fractures near the hip must be operated upon with expedition and in such a manner that the patient is out of bed next day.

Experience shows that the elderly both tolerate and respond well to operations and that, properly given, general anaesthesia does not cause a problem. After an anaesthetic, at which the anaesthetist is able to aspirate the mucus and secretions from the lungs, the elderly patients are often better than before the operation. This, combined with the activity of being up the next day, greatly enhances the outlook in general.

Many patients admitted after an injury have multiple physical ailments. A limited assessment of the general condition before the operation, which is then done as soon as reasonably possible, is better than delaying the operation for a full investigation which should be done afterwards. Then the necessary treatment of the other conditions that will have been found can be done at leisure without the patient having the extreme discomfort of the untreated fracture or the disadvantage of not being able to be up.

With age comes weakness; with loss of muscle power comes loss of bone strength; osteoporosis, particularly marked in women, is always present, and the longer the patient is in bed the greater the increase in osteoporosis from decubitus itself as well as from further loss of muscle tone. It is almost impossible to regain the power lost from several weeks in bed, and impossible if decubitus lasts for months. Because of this, rehabilitation (which includes the surgical procedure) has to achieve in the shortest possible time the activities of daily living so that the patient, out of bed, may dress, sit at table, walk to the toilet and become independent.

It is possible to sum up the aims of the rehabilitation of the elderly in the most important physical sign in geriatric orthopaedics which is to see the patient walk. Without walking the elderly person is certain to have lost full independence and a satisfactory quality of life.

On those occasions when it is necessary to leave an elderly patient to a wheelchair existence because rehabilitation to a greater level of independence is impossible (and this may not be because of the orthopaedic lesion, but from vascular disease, heart failure, chest disease or mental confusion), the decision for this must be taken only after considerable thought and discussion and must in no way be lightly made. It is, in essence, a confession of failure to rehabilitate the patient satisfactorily.

There is no detail of treatment too insignificant for consideration by the orthopaedic surgeon. The full, detailed and careful history and examination is nowhere more important than in being able to assess the problems and proper treatment of the patient, both from the general and from the local point of view. Before any decision can be made in regard to the surgery of the part affected, the patient and her circumstances must be fully considered. It is most important not only to know that the patient can do up her shoes or put on her stockings, but how many stairs there are at home, and with whom, if anyone, the patient lives. These, and the innumerable other big and small difficulties that beset each elderly patient, make it necessary to have a team to help manage all the problems that surround the proper and full treatment of an orthopaedic lesion that has occurred in an old person.

The team will include the medical social worker, the occupational therapist and physiotherapist, to investigate all aspects of the circumstances and present physical abilities of the patient, as well as the nursing and medical staff.

It is very important for the patients to know what is going on. Often deafness prevents them from hearing the remarks made and advice given, or at best, only part is understood. Slight confusion adds to this. The patient will respond far better to treatment if it is known what is happening, and why. Care taken in explaining the programme to the patient will always be rewarded by better progress.

Each patient must have a programme which must be known to all the team. Time, under no circumstances, is ever to be wasted and it is vital to have a ward round once a week attended by every member of the team whether this be in the geriatric orthopaedic unit or in the acute orthopaedic ward. Only in this way will the action of all be concerted, immediate and directed to the same goal. It will eliminate paper work such as requests for consultation or treatment because all members of the team make their own arrangements on the spot. Time is more vital in the treatment of the elderly patient than at any other age. Many have not long to live and do not wish to waste what time is left to them waiting for one or another member of the hospital staff to come to assess or advise with the consequent and ever recurring delays between each visit.

It is not uncommon to hear a surgeon remark that his hospital beds are blocked by elderly patients with fractured femora, as though this was the fault of the patient for being elderly; in fact it is criticism of the methods used which do not provide a satisfactory system of rehabilitation for the geriatric patients who are then unable to regain independence and go home.

It is always possible to organise a geriatric orthopaedic unit, even when there is apparently no space or bed available. The allocation of beds for such a unit, preferably in a geriatric ward, where both physician and surgeon could combine their responsibilities will soon show an overall saving of beds and, which is most important, greatly augment the facilities of rehabilitation to the consequent benefit of the patients who are then able to return home to an independent existence.

The nursing care of the geriatric patient, whether this be orthopaedic or medical, is in no way different to the nursing of any other patient but needs a higher concentration of nurses. This is because, in the orthopaedic ward, all elderly patients have to be up the day after operation; this does not apply to younger patients. Most elderly people after an operation need two people to help them out of bed and to walk; help is needed to go to the toilet, sometimes even to eat. Skin care requires far more attention than it does in the young patient, as do the bowels and the bladder. So it will be readily appreciated that a geriatric orthopaedic patient, if to be successfully rehabilitated in the shortest time, needs the highest calibre of nursing care with an establishment on the geriatric orthopaedic ward equal to that of an acute medical or surgical ward.

Geriatric Assessment

The problem of a major operation on an old person is often assumed to be far beyond the physical stamina of the patient concerned and is dismissed by the unreasonable assumption that the patient is not fit for such a procedure as, for example, a total hip replacement. This concept is entirely wrong and it is more important to consider whether the patient is fit enough to be denied the operation because, without it, the struggle against the pain and disability may well overtax the willpower of the patient who then becomes entirely dependent on others.

The disability caused by a hip or knee which is painful, stiff or unstable is tremendous and the danger of falling, because of the failure of the part concerned, means that the patient may be admitted for an emergency operation which could have been prevented by the elective operation done in good time. Further, the disability, even if not causing a fall, will deny the patient the full activity possible, the patient will become first house bound and later chair bound so that not only is there little pleasure in life but independence is lost.

Much can be done to improve an old person before operation, given a little time. Here the geriatrician can assess and determine the coexistent conditions and treat and give warning of them. The physiotherapist will not only instruct in exercises for the hip or knee, but will treat the chest and also, which is most important, assess with the occupational therapist the capabilities of the patient so that they may be known before operation. Of course there are many octogenarians who are very fit and appear to need no assessment but even in this group a careful examination will reveal, every so often, some potential hazard whether it be from a hiatus hernia or incipient cardiac ischaemia.

It is because of this absolute necessity of involving the Geriatric Department in the care of the elderly patient both before and after operation that Chapter 2 deals with this aspect of geriatric orthopaedics. Without such assistance the orthopaedic surgeon would be unable to manage the quick rehabilitation of his patients, whether elective or emergency.

Geriatric Anaesthesia

Elderly patients are never too old for operation, nor do they take a general anaesthetic badly. These are myths easily dispelled by a competent anaesthetist who understands the special problems and assesses the patients beforehand. It is true to say that nowhere is an old person safer than in the hands of the anaesthetist on the operation table.

The anaesthetist has two roles to play in the treatment of the geriatric orthopaedic patient: first resuscitation after an emergency admission and, second, the care of the patient during anaesthesia. Both need adjustment of the applications of the principles of anaesthesia; these are dealt with in Chapters 3 and 4 in which considerable detail in treatment is given because it is important to dispel any anxiety about operating upon the very old under a general anaesthetic. The anaesthetist will know that after an emergency admission early operation is indicated so he will resuscitate the patient with all expedition, but not without proper consideration. Sometimes there are definite indications for postponing operation for a short while, but it is important to remember that it is unusual for an elderly patient to improve with delay after an accident and in the presence of a painful fracture. Two of the most important exceptions are untreated heart failure and untreated diabetes but neither need delay the patient more than a day or so provided the physicians concerned also understand the need for speed. Sometimes hypothermia or severe dehydration has to be corrected before operation, but again this does not take long.

The experienced anaesthetist will also recognise that once a fracture has been fixed and pain relieved, most patients improve remarkably. This means that even if a patient appears to be dying anaesthesia is not necessarily contra-indicated because the wellbeing of the patient is served best by dispelling a painful lesion.

Death

Old people know that their life span is limited. It is the young person who feels immortal in this life, but the elderly are often impatient with the sufferings of this world and are ready for the next. This does not alter the oldest principle of medicine, that one should heal the sick. An old person, however ill, should be treated in the best possible way which must, of necessity, have kindness included in the treatment.

Thus, because an old lady, ill and frail, is admitted with a fracture near the hip, she should not be abandoned as too ill to treat, or worse, too old. Only if moribund should operation be deferred, with suitable treatment to ease the pain.

Apart from this, often such a patient makes some recovery, even if it is merely that she does not die. Then operation is indicated because it is unlikely that the anaesthetic will cause death and it is possible that, after the operation, the patient will improve and even regain independence. The operation is not done to save life but to give it a better quality while it lasts. To be allowed to lie in a ward for many days or weeks dying with an untreated fracture near the hip is poor medicine.

Rheumatoid Arthritis

The ravages that rheumatoid arthritis produces in the joints of the elderly give it a special place in geriatric orthopaedics. It has been found, and is of general experience, that with increasing age there is an increasing rate of rheumatoid arthritis.

Old people with rheumatoid arthritis need special help and continued observation because they must not be allowed to become so crippled that they are no longer able to manage the activities of daily living. Once they have lost their independence surgical rehabilitation is much more difficult because of the general involvement of joints with, at the same time, the same number of other ailments that beset any old person. Thus it is important to operate on a patient with rheumatoid arthritis long before the condition has reached so deplorable a state that function is lost. The geriatric rheumatoid patient also has weakness of old age compounded by the muscular weakness associated with the disease, even if peripheral neuritis is not present. Further, rheumatoid arthritis alone, but specially if treated by steroid drugs, may have produced osteoporosis to a greater amount than is usual for the particular age group concerned. Therefore it is important for the rheumato-logist to understand the surgical problems of his patients because he is the best person to prepare a patient with rheumatoid arthritis for operation. This is best done in the rheumatology ward and the patient transferred to the orthopaedic ward merely for the operation and returned again afterwards. Either way the surgery takes its proper place in the care of the rheumatoid and geriatric patient; that is, being an incident in the overall programme of treatment.

Finally, to achieve the understanding necessary between the two specialists it is essential to have combined clinics where patients can be seen together not only before operation, but afterwards so that the effect of the surgical results can be reviewed.

Orthopaedics in the Elderly

There are some surgical procedures for the elderly that differ in technique from that done in the younger patient, but apart from this, most of the surgery described here is to emphasise its place in the rehabilitation of the elderly. Those techniques specially applicable will be described in detail even though the principle of the operation remains the same, because a rigid adherence to the operative technique used on the younger patient may not be in the best interests of the older person. A simple example is in the internal fixation of the fractured shaft of femur; in the elderly there is no contra-indication to approaching the femoral shaft through the knee and inserting an intra-medullary rod with greater expedition and care than with the accepted methods used on young patients.

The advantages of varying the technique of operation in an old person must give positive advantages; whether it be to allow the patient to walk sooner or merely to lessen the time and blood loss at operation. The price to be paid for the advantages, which would not be acceptable in the young, might be a later secondary arthritis or other disability which, in the elderly, has insufficient time to appear. The principles of fracture treatment are the same for any age but the different ways in which the principles are applied will be dealt with fully. It is most important, when operating on an elderly patient, to obviate the fracture as soon as possible especially if it confines the patient to bed.

The indications for internal fixation of a fracture in a geriatric patient are quite different from those in youth and are indeed reversed. It is necessary to have a definite indication not to operate in an old and feeble patient for otherwise rehabilitation will be greatly hindered.

Most of the elective operations for arthritis are in the elderly and here joint replacement has its greatest part to play. It is not possible to describe all the methods and therefore only those for which there has been considerable experience at Hastings will be described. There are, indeed, some forms of replacement which are contra-indicated for the elderly patient who requires the utmost stability and immediate return to function as part of the indication for surgery. In this respect a knee replacement which needs a cast for several weeks thereafter should not be used. Only those methods which will allow the patient to walk the next day unimpeded by splintage may be used. The same applies to the hip joint. No method should be used which does not allow the patient to be out of bed the next day.

After all orthopaedic procedures on an old person it is wrong to attempt to achieve a range of movement or an activity which is not necessary for the wellbeing of the patient. After a total hip replacement, provided the patient can do all those things she wishes to do including all the activities of daily living, and providing she can find no fault herself with the hip, the fact that it will not achieve the same range of movement as in a young adult is immaterial. It is wrong to subject such a patient to continued and unnecessary treatment to try to achieve that range.

Pathological Fractures

It is in the elderly that most pathological fractures occur. These may be secondary to Paget's disease or malignancy and once the fracture has occurred it must be dealt with like any other fracture, that is, internally fixed so that the fracture is obviated. This allows the radiotherapy to be given to the patient in comfort and from any direction needed. No ill effects are occasioned by the metal within the patient.

It is important to treat all pathological lesions as soon as possible because it is unlikely that the general condition will improve with delay. It is particularly important when the illness is nearing a terminal stage; then a successful operation will determine the quality of existence for the limited time left to the patient.

To keep a patient in the discomfort of a large plaster cast in hospital while the radiotherapist gives treatment is wrong when, after a suitable operation, she could be independent and at home having the treatment as an out-patient. It is far better, and makes radiotherapy far easier, if a determined orthopaedic attack is made and the lesion dealt with to preserve this independence. Never should a patient with painful secondaries be considered too ill to be operated upon, assuming there is a suitable method of treatment available, because the alternative is heavy sedation until death. The risk of operation may seem great, but the prize of a few days or weeks of lucidity is always worth while and conforms to the best interests of good medicine.

An impending pathological fracture should be treated before the fracture occurs; it is then simple and quick; it prevents a catastrophe and cures the pain.

Paraplegia from metastatic deposits is one of the greatest tragedies that can occur to old people. At once it deprives them of independence and condemns them to a lingering death in circumstances that are an insult to the dignity of death. Even returning home to die is usually impossible. Therefore a determined surgical attack is indicated and may often give a new, if short, lease of life. However, the mortality of operation is high. The orthopaedic surgeon with a proper appreciation of life will carry a heavy mortality rate for this operation; it is inevitable, but he will have grateful patients and grateful relatives who will know that all has been done that could be done.

Amputations

Many old people are confined to bed after amputations because there is no suitable method of getting them on to an early walking programme because the particular hospital is not adjacent or attached to a limb fitting centre. To obtain an artificial limb the patient has to visit the limb fitting centre. For many patients this is too far, the journey too tiring and the delays too exorbitant.

Without an early walking aid the patient may be able to sit out of bed and hobble a step or two with a pair of crutches if they are not mentally confused or otherwise too decrepit but it is a poor substitute for proper walking. Every patient who has an amputation should be provided with an early walking aid at the earliest possible moment. It is not right to wait six weeks for a pylon. At Hastings a system of early walking has been in operation for many years and has proved safe and reliable. No amputee should be subjected to the loss of a high percentage of the enjoyment of her remaining life by failure to provide early walking facilities; one third of geriatric amputees die within a year, and another third within a further two years of amputation. Often without early walking many months may pass before independence is achieved. The failure to walk may also debilitate the patient and ultimately rehabilitation on to a definitive limb is at best difficult or at the worst impossible.

Osteoporosis

The ever continuing arguments about the cause and treatment of osteoporosis have, as yet, produced no cure and no prevention. A long experience with geriatric orthopaedic surgery shows that, whatever the amount of bone may be in any particular part, provided it can be allowed to join together when broken, it will do so and do so very well indeed. There is no fear of non-union because of osteoporosis. Nor need there be any fear of doing any other procedure, provided the technique is satisfactory and adjusted to the condition of the bone.

One point that will emerge is that, after a successful arthroplasty of a joint that has hindered the activity of an old person, there is a very real possibility of a stress fracture occurring in the same or the opposite limb. This is because the level of activity before the operation needed little muscular tone or strength; the rapid, if not actually sudden, return to activity will allow the muscles to regain their strength much faster than does the bone. Hence power and usage are so increased that the bone, already osteoporotic from age, with further osteoporosis from disuse, will have insufficient strength and break from the stresses imposed upon it.

Stress Fractures

Any age group can have special stress fractures but the elderly share, paradoxically, many of the same patterns of this condition as do children.

The most important result of a stress fracture in the elderly is a complete fracture. Although this can occur in youth it is more common in later life. Therefore any stress fracture must be considered carefully, and in certain circumstances prophylactic internal fixation should be done.

Some fractures of the neck of the femur and some tibial fractures are caused by a stress fracture becoming complete, sometimes with no injury, sometimes with some trivial jar. A careful history and good radiology will usually prove that this was the case.

The minutiae of treatment will not be described in this book unless they are different from those normally accepted. Then the difference will be emphasised so that the philosophy and reasoning causing the change in method will be fully understood.

Geriatric patients are dignified in their acceptance of the inevitable end and do not ask for longevity but they do ask for a quality of life that is satisfactory. Often this is synonymous with a return of function which, in the elderly, is return to independence.

2

Medical Care in Geriatric Orthopaedics

R. E. IRVINE and T. M. STROUTHIDIS

The objective of surgery in old age is not always to save life. More often, particularly in orthopaedics, it is to improve the quality of living, to relieve pain, to increase mobility and to enable the patient to enjoy the greatest possible degree of independence. It is often necessary to be content with modest goals. Sometimes it may be enough to relieve pain and make nursing easier.

Advances in anaesthesia and surgical technique have made the operation itself perhaps the safest period in the patient's illness, so that the outcome depends not only on the local lesion but on the state of the patient as a whole. In old people an operation is often complicated by co-existing medical problems and by the failure of a system other than that which is being subjected to surgery. The older the patient the more important and the more numerous become the complications of pre-existing illness. Moreover the patient's physiological age is often very different from her chronological age. A geriatric physician is trained to assess the patient as a whole, taking account of the medical, psychological and social factors which, in addition to operative technique, determine the outcome of surgery.

In emergency surgery the physician's role before operation may be confined to the management of acute cardiac failure, unstable diabetes and electrolyte disturbances. The more detailed investigation of the patient is better left until after the emergency, usually a fracture, has been treated. In elective surgery on the other hand the geriatrician can contribute to a full assessment of the patient so that she comes to the operation table in the best possible condition.

The Cause of the Fracture

If the patient has sustained a fracture (and this is the commonest reason for involving the geriatric physician) it is important to determine the cause. This is usually from a fall but there are some patients in whom the lesion is a stress fracture. Stress fractures may manifest themselves by increasing pain in one hip without a fall or by a sudden pain with a feeling of something giving way in the hip preceding a fall. A few other patients sustain a pathological fracture involving a bone weakened by neoplastic disease.

The severity of the injury necessary to produce a fracture declines with age because the bones become more fragile. The fragility appears to be selective and affects mainly the proximal femur, the proximal humerus, the distal radius, the vertebral bodies and finally the distal femur. The risk of fracture begins to increase from the time of the menopause and doubles with every five years after the age of 60.

The principal reason lies in the bone loss, or osteoporosis, which occurs with ageing. It affects both sexes but is of greater clinical importance in women. Both men and women lose bone steadily from the age of 25, but women begin life with less bone, and their bone loss accelerates after the menopause. They also outnumber men by two to one in older age groups.

One of the unsolved problems of osteoporosis, however, is that although ageing is the most important factor, it is not the only one. At least three diseases, rheumatoid arthritis, thyrotoxicosis and Cushing's syndrome increase the loss of bone. So do bed rest, immobilisation and treatment with corticosteroids. These must, as far as possible, be avoided in the management of illness in old people. No treatment for osteoporosis is of proven value. Oestrogens, androgens, anabolic steroids, fluoride, calcium and calcitonin have all had their advocates. Some will reverse a negative calcium balance and decrease the excretion of hydroxyproline. None have been shown to increase the volume or density of bone.

Another bone disease known to increase the risk of fractures is osteomalacia, caused by the lack of vitamin D. Dietary deficiency and lack of exposure to sunlight are the main causes, but partial gastrectomy, malabsorption syndromes and prolonged treatment with anticonvulsants are also known to predispose to osteomalacia. The newly formed preosteal tissue, osteoid, fails to calcify. The serum levels of calcium and phosphate are often but not invariably reduced. The serum alkaline phosphatase level is usually raised.

Until recently only severe cases, characterised by bone pain, pseudo fractures (Looser's zones) and proximal muscle weakness have been recognised. Now, however, routine bone biopsies of the iliac crest in patients with femoral neck fractures have revealed that lesser degrees of osteomalacia are far more common than was previously recognised. Some degree of osteomalacia may be present in as many as a quarter of all women with femoral neck fractures, and an even higher proportion of men.

Facilities for bone biopsy are not available to us at Hastings. Where there is biochemical evidence of osteomalacia, our practice is to give calciferol 50 000 units (1.25 milligrams) daily for two weeks. Thereafter these patients, like all others who have sustained a fracture, are given one tablet daily of calcium and vitamin D (B.P.C.) or one capsule of vitamins A and D (B.P.C.). The first contains 500 and the second 450 units of vitamin D. Patients are urged to take this medication indefinitely and to expose themselves to sunlight whenever possible.

The incidence of Paget's disease increases steadily with age and affects one in ten of those over 90. It may contribute to a fracture, which is usually obvious from the radiographs. Usually no medical treatment is required, but if there is bone pain, this can be greatly helped by injections of calcitonin. The synthetic salmon calcitonin, Calsynar, is the most convenient medication and the dose is from 50 units three times a week to 100 units daily by subcutaneous or intramuscular injection. Daily injections, apart from the inconvenience to the patient, cost £30 per week, so it is important to ensure that the patient's pain is, in fact, caused by the Paget's disease and not by an associated osteoarthritis. The least dose that is effective should be used and for as short a time as possible. Treatment for 18 days may relieve pain for more than a year.

In old age multiple pathology is the rule; this means that any one disorder of bone does not necessarily exclude others and it is to be expected that many disorders may occur together in one patient.

The Cause of the Fall

The commonest fall to cause a fracture is an ordinary trip or stumble, usually in the home. A loose mat, a missed step, an unstable hand hold and poor lighting are common factors in the environment. Poor eyesight and increasing instability of walking with advancing age are common predisposing factors in these patients. In a few, sudden head movements, looking upwards or turning the head to the side may cause acute ischaemia of the brain stem and thus provoke a fall. A common cause is a drop attack, in which the patient's legs suddenly give way so that she falls to the ground without warning and without loss of consciousness. The origin of these attacks is still disputed but they are probably related to cervical spondylosis and vertebro-basilar ischaemia. They are often controlled if the patient wears a cervical collar.

The fall is often associated with previous cerebro-vascular disease or disorders such as Parkinsonism which impair the righting reflexes of the patient. Joint disease, unless accompanied by neurological impairment, is not an important factor.

About one in ten of all falls occur at night when the patient gets out of bed to go to the lavatory or to use a bedside commode. Usually it is difficult to ascertain what actually has happened because the patient is often half asleep, but the sudden change from recumbency to the erect position suggests the possibility of postural hypotension. Sleeping tablets, tranquillisers, anti-depressants and diuretics are all known to predispose to postural hypotension and may be additional factors. Acute syncope from cardiac causes such as paroxysmal tachycardia or heart block can be suspected from the pulse and from the cardiogram. Epilepsy as a cause of fracture is suggested by the previous history.

Complications after Operation

Medical complications occurring after operation are the concern of the geriatric physician. It is because of the frequency and seriousness of these complications that the more ill patients are transferred from the acute orthopaedic wards to the special unit, described in Chapter 14.

CONFUSION

Confusion is a common reaction of the aged to the stress of an operation. The anaesthetic and surgery are probably contributory especially if there has been a fall in blood pressure with diminished cerebral perfusion during the period of recovery, which is to be avoided by all methods possible as described in Chapter 3; but unless the patient was mentally disturbed before admission, such confusion is seldom of great importance and usually clears within a few days. It is important to talk to the patient, to explain where she is, what has happened to her and what is going to happen. If possible she should not be left in darkness. It is important to make sure that she is not lying in a wet bed or suffering from the discomfort of urinary retention which is so often secondary to faecal impaction. It may help to give the patient a cup of tea, or, sometimes, a stronger stimulant.

If she remains restless and noisy, however, a tranquilliser will be necessary, for example chlorpromazine (Largactil) 25 to 50 milligrams by mouth, perhaps supplemented with a hypnotic such as chlormethiazole 500 to 1000 milligrams as a capsule or as a syrup. If the patient will not take medication by mouth then 50 milligrams of chlorpromazine or 5 milligrams of haloperidol (Serenace) may be injected intramuscularly. Paraldehyde must be avoided.

Tranquillisers should not be repeated more often than is absolutely necessary. Heavy sedation is likely to increase the risk of pressure sores, venous thrombosis, dehydration and pneumonia. An agitated patient is often made worse if she is restrained in bed with safety sides and these should be avoided wherever possible. If she is in an adjustable height bed it should be in the low position so that she is less likely to injure herself if she gets out of bed. It is better to let her get up into a chair and to go to the lavatory than to imprison her behind bars in bed.

INCONTINENCE OF URINE

Incontinence of urine is often associated with confusion and with the enforced immobility of the early period after operation. It occurs in about half of all old women with a femoral neck fractūre and often justifies the use of a catheter draining to a leg bag for the first few days. Most patients regain control of the bladder within a short time but about one third remain incontinent for much longer. The best way to restore the patient's continence is to encourage mobility and to offer the chance of walking to the lavatory as soon as possible: preferably the latter should be suitably placed but if this is difficult, as it is in many old buildings not designed for geriatric patients, then a bedside commode is a suitable alternative. As far as possible the bedpan should be avoided. Disposable incontinence pads are of value and an insurance against wet sheets, provided that the large size is used. They should be placed in the bed with the bonded edges running across and not along the bed. Kanga pants offer some additional protection, particularly for women, but may lead to skin soreness if worn day and night. For men, it is easy to leave a bottle by the bed. In patients who remain incontinent after the first few days it is worth trying anticholinergic drugs such as emepronium bromide (Cetiprin) 200 milligrams or flavoxate (Urispas) 200 milligrams, each three times a day. In women the oestrogenic substance, quinoestradol (Pentovis) 1000 milligrams daily for two or three weeks is worth a trial.

INCONTINENCE OF FAECES

Incontinence of faeces is usually caused by faecal retention with overflow. When an old person is faecally incontinent, this should always be assumed to be the case until proved otherwise. A finger inserted into the rectum will reveal that it is loaded, usually with pultaceous, but occasionally with very hard faeces which have a characteristically pungent odour. It is not difficult to remove some of the faeces manually and a series of phosphate enemas (B.P.C.) are then given to clear the bowel. If the faeces have become very hard an arachis oil retention enema may be necessary. Purgatives given by mouth are not effective and may cause griping. Once faecal retention has occurred it is necessary to give repeated enemas until the bowel is clear. Daily enemas are best unless they overtax the patient's strength, when they may be given every two or three days.

Once the bowel is clear it is important to preserve its function by giving the patient two dessertspoonsful of bran each day with porridge, cereal or soup. This may be supplemented by a faecal softener such as Dioctyl Forte 100 milligrams three times a day, or by a laxative such as Senokot.

PRESSURE SORES

A fracture of the proximal femur used to be called the unsolved fracture. Now it has a good solution. The unsolved problem in elderly patients with fractured femora has now become the pressure sore. Pressure sores occur in one third of all patients with fractures of the proximal femur, a much higher incidence than is found in the geriatric patients generally. The seeds are probably sown in the period of immobility between the occurrence of the fracture and its surgical fixation.

Pressure sores are of two kinds, superficial and deep. Superficial sores are painful and associated with maceration of the skin by urine and by friction with the bed linen. Most often they occur over the sacrum and buttocks. Fortunately they heal quickly once the patient regains mobility.

Deep sores are less common, but much more serious. They occur in about ten per cent of patients. A common site is the heel of the side of the fracture but sores may occur over the sacrum, ischia or the trochanters. They are caused by prolonged pressure which obliterates the blood supply and leads to deep tissue necrosis. A deep sore is preceded by a short period when the threatened tissues feel indurated. There is then an eruption from within outwards and bone is rapidly exposed. Deep sores take months to heal, if they heal at all. They become infected, impair the patient's general health and may contribute to her death. At the very least they prolong the stay in hospital by many months.

Prevention

The best treatment for pressure sores is to prevent them. This advice is easy to give but very difficult to achieve in practice with the resources available in most hospitals.

The most important predisposing factor is immobility and the patient with a recent fracture of the femur, not yet fixed, is at very high risk. Two hourly turning is the secret of pressure sore prevention, but in the period between the fracture and the operation, this is painful and may well have to be omitted. Moreover certain fractures are so painful that traction is necessary and this is incompatible with turning. The only nursing aid which dispenses with the need for two hourly turning is the water bed. If the patient lies on a water bed, her weight is evenly distributed and pressure over bony prominences is reduced. The pressure on the heels and sacrum for example is 20 to 25 millimetres of mercury compared with 35 to 40 millimetres of mercury on a foam mattress or a Ripple bed and 200 millimetres of mercury on an operating table. The capillary blood pressure is 27 millimetres of mercury but when a patient is lying on a water bed the blood supply to her skin is still maintained even at points of greatest pressure. Water beds have many disadvantages however. They are heavy and difficult to move. They are expensive. They are of fixed height and make it difficult for the patient to get in and out. It is hard to use a bedpan. Most importantly the water temperature must be electrically maintained at a constant level and the thermostats often go wrong. Nevertheless we believe that before operation a patient with femoral fractures should be nursed on a water bed.

A subsidiary factor contributing to pressure sores before operation is incontinence. Men confined to bed can manage with a bottle, but for women there is an indication for a self retaining catheter.

After operation the principle is to get the patient moving as soon as possible. A patient who is in good physical condition, fully alert in mind, continent, able to walk and to move freely about the bed will not get a pressure sore. On the other hand a patient who is in poor physical condition, mentally impaired, inactive, immobile and doubly incontinent is very likely to develop a sore. A scoring system devised by Norton, McLaren and Exton Smith (1975) quantifies the risk and enables those most likely to develop sores to be identified. The patient is assigned a mark from nought to three for each of the five points mentioned above. When these are added together they create a scale from zero when all is favourable to 15 when all is as bad as can be. Experience shows that patients whose scores are eight or more are at risk for pressure sores and need special attention (Fig. 1). Those deemed to be at risk should be nursed on a water bed without two hourly turning or on a large celled Ripple mattress with two hourly turning. It is reasonable to control incontinence with a catheter for a few days. Medical complications must be dealt with and this will often improve the patient's physical and mental state, allowing mobilisation to begin. The patient's score should be regularly reviewed so that special nursing can be discontinued as soon as possible. Scoring takes only half a minute to do, but special nursing with two hourly turning is very expensive in nursing time.

When a patient acquires a deep sore, it is usually because what should have been done was left undone. This is easy to understand, particularly at night when it is hard to provide sufficient nurses to ensure continued two hourly turning. A deep pressure sore should not be shrugged off or accepted, however. Each time one occurs, it should be the subject of a discussion between the medical and nursing staff to try to discover what went wrong and how their practice could be improved.

Treatment

A superficial sore requires only a dry dressing and will heal if the patient becomes mobile. If there is incontinence there is always a danger that the dressing will become wet and act as a urinary poultice thus increasing the damage to the skin. For this reason sores around the buttocks and sacrum are often left uncovered. It is of course possible to keep the patient dry by catheterisation, but every day on a catheter is a day lost in the rehabilitation of the bladder. Some compromise is necessary, but in general it is a mistake to allow the interests of the local lesion to take precedence over the rehabilitation of the patient as a whole.

A patient with a deep sore must be nursed on a water bed, but should be up and walking whenever this is possible. No sore will begin to heal while slough and eschar are still present and these must be removed with forceps and scissors as opportunity permits. Infected sores are seldom helped by local or systemic antibiotics, but eusol and paraffin are still the most useful dressings. Deep sores must be kept covered to lessen the loss of fluid and protein.

It is also important to attend to the patient's general condition. The

EAST SUSSEX AREA HEALTH AUTHORITY
HASTINGS HEALTH DISTRICT

PRESSURE SORE RISK AND PROGRESS CHART

.... Hospital

Name   Age :   No.

Scoring System. Total score of 8 or more indicates a risk of pressure sores

A.	Physical State	Good............0	Fair............1	Poor............2	V. Bad 3
B.	Mental State	Good............0	Apathetic 1	Confused 2	Stuporous 3
C.	Activity	Ambulant 0	Walk/Help 1	Chairfast 2	Bedfast 3
D.	Mobility	Full 0	Sl. Limited 1	V. Limited 2	Immobile 3
E.	Incontinence	None............0	Occasional 1	Usual/Ur. 2	Double 3

Date	A	B	C	D	E	Total	Remarks

FIG. 1 The chart used to assess the risk of pressure sores in geriatric patients.

haemoglobin and serum protein levels must be maintained as well as is possible. Blood transfusion may be necessary together with a high protein diet. Vitamin C 500 milligrams twice daily and zinc sulphate capsules 220 milligrams three times daily have been shown to help the healing of sores.

The healing of the sore may be charted by serial photographs or more simply, by measuring the longest diameter of the sore at weekly intervals.

THROMBOEMBOLISM

Another difficult problem is thromboembolism and the use of anticoagulants. We prefer not to use anticoagulants routinely because they can cause haematomata and in our view add to the complications of surgery. We prefer to rely on early mobilisation although we are aware that it is not completely effective. About five per cent of our patients develop clinically obvious venous thromboses requiring anticoagulant treatment. The number of deaths from pulmonary embolism is about 1.5%.

On the other hand it is known from radioactive fibrinogen studies that 75% of those with a fractured neck of femur have deep vein thromboses. Most of these are not detectable clinically and resolve spontaneously. Some authors report a high degree of correlation between the results of radioactive fibrinogen scanning and venography, but others find that only about half the thromboses detected by radioactive scanning are confirmed at venography. Even when there is leg swelling, clinically suggestive of deep vein thrombosis, venographic confirmation of the diagnosis is lacking in 25% of patients. It has been suggested that a combination of operative trauma and immobility causes inadequate action of the muscle pump and increased vascular permeability leading to oedema and extravasation of fibrin into the tissues. This remains an unsolved problem.

Medical Assessment

The problems so far considered arise either before operation or in the first few days afterwards. About a week after operation, or sooner if she is very ill, the patient may come to the orthopaedic geriatric unit where a full medical assessment is undertaken. To obtain a good history the doctor should not only talk to the patient but should try to meet some of her relatives and friends, and this is much easier when the ward has open visiting; they can often explain better than the patient what was her pattern of life before the injury. Old people are capable of a great deal of self deception and will often present a much rosier account of their social circumstances and activities than the facts justify. It is important to learn how the patient has been living and what she could do before the fracture. The physician is as much concerned with function as with traditional diagnosis. Has the patient been able to go out or was she housebound? Can she cook and do housework or does she need home help? Is she still living in her own home or is she now needing some form of residential care with members of her family or in an institution? Is she mentally clear or is she forgetful? Is she of independent personality or is she someone who has always made demands on others? Such questions will reveal the patient's previous degree of dependence. The information will be of great importance in planning her rehabilitation and resettlement. The more a patient's functional capacity is impaired the more important it becomes to identify underlying medical factors and to understand her personality. After obtaining as full a history as possible careful clinical examination follows. This must include an assessment of the patient's mental state. Her sight and hearing must be considered so that everything is done to maintain her powers of communication. It is important to look for any neurological abnormality and for evidence of joint disease which may impede progress. The need for chiropody should be assessed. The patient should be carefully examined for pressure sores, which are easily missed unless she is turned on her side and the buttocks and heels carefully inspected. Routine investigations include radiography of the chest and of the injured part, an electrocardiogram, haematological investigations and an assessment of the blood levels of urea, electrolytes, sugar, calcium, phosphorus, alkaline phosphatase, and plasma proteins with an electrophoretic strip. A midstream specimen of urine should be examined in men. In women a specimen taken with a short catheter attached to a bag, the Alexa female specimen set, is better.

MENTAL STATE
An indispensable part of the examination is an assessment of the patient's mental state. Ten per cent of the population over 65 show some degree of mental impairment and in half of these it is severe. Over the age of 80 mental impairment is present in one out of five of the population. Because many of these also have physical infirmities it is usual in the geriatric unit to find that at least half the patients admitted are mentally impaired. Mental impairment, or brain failure as it is now sometimes called, shortens the expectation of life and makes it harder for the patient to participate in her own rehabilitation.

In the Hastings geriatric unit a simple ten point questionnaire devised by Dr. Leslie Wilson of Aberdeen has been found very convenient. It takes only a few minutes to administer and can be used on every patient capable of speaking. The questions asked are shown in Table I. A normal old person can answer correctly eight questions out of ten. The results are remarkably reproduceable provided that the patient is in a stable state emotionally. When a patient has a low score at first testing and improves later this normally indicates the clearing of a temporary confusional state.

MOOD
It is important also to assess the patient's mood. Anxiety and depression are

Table I

ABERDEEN MENTAL STATUS QUESTIONNAIRE

1. What is this town?	6. What year were you born?
2. What month were you born?	7. Who is the Prime Minister?
3. What is this place?	8. What year is it now?
4. What is your age?	9. What is the date to-day?
5. What is this month?	10. Who was the last Prime Minister?

even more common than mental impairment in the elderly population and a patient who has recently sustained a fracture and undergone a major operation with a transfer from one hospital to another may be justifiably apprehensive. Much can be done to set the patient at ease by a kindly and welcoming atmosphere, but those who are most afflicted may need a tranquilliser or antidepressant before they are able to participate effectively in their rehabilitation. The recognition of depressive illness in the elderly is difficult because they are exposed to so many unfavourable social factors, isolation, bereavement, poverty and physical illness which might make anyone dejected. The last thing of which the patient is likely to complain is depression in so many words. It is more likely that she will show a lack of energy, a lack of interest or a preoccupation with physical complaints. She may be agitated or apathetic. Disturbed sleep, a good sign of depression in younger people, is less reliable in the elderly since many of them are used to waking several times at night. In any case it is hard to sleep well in a hospital ward. One useful question to ask is: "In spite of all that has happened to you, do you still find life worth living?".

CIRCULATORY SYSTEM

Diseases of the heart and circulation are found in up to 50% of elderly orthopaedic patients. Sometimes they provide the reason for the fall which led to the fracture. A careful clinical examination must include not only the heart, lungs and blood pressure but also the pulses in the legs and feet. It should be supplemented routinely by a chest radiograph and an electrocardiogram. The chest radiograph is the only reliable way of estimating heart size. The larger the heart the poorer the prognosis in all forms of heart disease. It is also not widely appreciated that a normal sized heart virtually excludes a diagnosis of congestive cardiac failure. The electrocardiogram may reveal evidence of recent or old cardiac infarction, of atrial fibrillation, or of some other disturbance of heart rhythm, including heart block, which may lead to syncope and falls.

Oedema of the legs is associated in every doctor's mind with congestive cardiac failure but this state is over diagnosed in old age. In the elderly oedema of the legs is more often caused by venous insufficiency, the result of prolonged inactivity or previous thrombophlebitis and varicose veins. It should never by itself be regarded as a sign of cardiac failure. Sacral oedema on the other hand is a reliable sign of cardiac failure, as are gallop rhythm and raised jugular venous pressure. An important sign of cardiac failure in the elderly is mental confusion, particularly if this is of sudden onset.

It is important to consider the cause of congestive cardiac failure if this is diagnosed. The commonest underlying pathology is ischaemic heart disease and failure may be provoked by a cardiac infarction, which is often painless, or by the onset of dysrhythmia. Other common causes include respiratory infection and repeated pulmonary emboli. Mitral and aortic valve disease is occasionally found in the elderly and so is sub-acute bacterial endocarditis. Rapid atrial fibrillation with or without failure should always suggest the possibility of thyrotoxicosis and the absence of a goitre does not exclude thyroid disease. Heart failure may also be iatrogenic, the result of over enthusiastic transfusion with blood or fluids or the administration of fluid retaining drugs such as oestrogens. Heart failure in old age usually responds well to treatment. Where there is atrial fibrillation digoxin is essential but the loading dose need not exceed 0.25 milligrams by mouth. After a few days the daily maintenance dose can be reduced to 0.0625 milligrams, as one Lanoxin-PG tablet. The most important drugs in cardiac failure are the diuretics. In emergency, intravenous frusemide (Lasix) 20 to 80 milligrams or bumetanide (Burinex) 1 milligram is very useful and if the patient has just sustained a fracture she should be catheterised so that the urine can be passed without painful movements. In men the introduction of a catheter has an additional advantage in that it avoids a common risk of diuretic treatment, acute retention of urine. Thiazide diuretics must be supplemented with potassium by mouth. Even in slow release preparations potassium is not without its problems, particularly that of dyspepsia. In milder cases there is a good indication for the use of a tablet combining a thiazide and a potassium retaining diuretic such as triamterine (Diazide, Dytide) or amiloride (Moduretic). Provided the precipitating cause of the failure can be controlled it is often unnecessary to continue cardiac therapy indefinitely. It is always worth seeing from time to time if the old person can do without her drugs.

HEART BLOCK

If the patient has heart block and a Stokes Adams attack has led to the fall the early introduction of a pacemaker will lead to a dramatic improvement.

POSTURAL HYPOTENSION

Postural hypotension is a common problem in the elderly and may interfere with rehabilitation after a fracture. In the normal subject vascular reflexes keep the blood pressure at the same level whether she is lying or standing. In the elderly patient with postural hypotension the blood pressure is normal when she is lying but falls to low levels when she stands. In severe cases it may be followed immediately by syncope. More often, however, the patient who, while lying in bed or sitting in a chair, seems well enough suddenly loses interest, goes silent, begins to sweat and looks ill when she stands up. A blood pressure reading will show a fall in blood pressure of perhaps 60 to 100 millimetres of mercury. The symptom has a number of causes which are not mutually exclusive. These include prolonged recumbency, a fall in cardiac output, as may happen after an infarction or after the administration of diuretics which reduce the blood volume, and interference with autonomic reflexes by antidepressants and phenothiazine tranquillisers. Occasionally the cause is autonomic neuropathy due to diabetes. Postural hypotension usually responds readily to treatment. The first step is to withdraw any offending drugs. The next is to re-educate the patient to assume the erect position. A tilting chair is useful to this end. A third measure is to support the legs with crepe bandages, Tubigrip or elastic stockings. It is very important that the physiotherapists are aware of this condition which may manifest itself most clearly during early attempts at standing and walking. It is quite often overlooked because doctors are reluctant to take the time required to measure the patient's blood pressure lying and standing.

NERVOUS SYSTEM

In at least a quarter of the patients with a fractured femur there is evidence of underlying neurological disease and the physician must look for it carefully. The most common are the features of a stroke, with signs of a hemiparesis, ataxia and speech disturbance and extensor plantar responses. The mask like faces of Parkinsonism with cogwheel rigidity and dyskinesia may also be obvious. Some patients show more bizarre disturbances of movement. A few have evidence of peripheral neuropathy.

Even in a patient with no obvious physical signs, warning of cerebro-vascular disease may be given by a history of transient cerebral ischaemic episodes with brief periods of confusion, dysphasia, dysarthria, dysphagia, paresis or visual disturbance. After such an incident relatives may comment that the old person has aged suddenly.

At present drugs play little part in the treatment of an old person with a stroke. Management is mainly a matter of rehabilitation and encouragement. There is some evidence, however, that regular aspirin in a dose of 300 milligrams daily reduces platelet adhesiveness and possibly the incidence of transient ischaemic attacks. Since we have no other drug to offer it is reasonable for any person who has had a stroke and fears another to take aspirin provided it does not upset her.

Parkinsonism is a regular cause of falls and fractures and it manifests itself somewhat differently in the elderly. Marked degrees of tremor are uncommon in old age. The main physical signs are rigidity and dyskinesia. Sometimes the voice may be affected and the patient may dribble because of difficulty in swallowing saliva. Parkinsonism in the elderly is often accompanied by mental impairment. Sometimes also there is peculiarly obstinate constipation. It is important to recognise Parkinsonism because it usually responds well to treatment. Levodopa, preferably with a dopa-decarboxylase inhibitor as in Sinemet and Madopar is often very effective. The elderly need smaller doses than the young and seldom require more than 3 grams of Levodopa or three tablets daily of Sinemet or Madopar. The new tablet of Sinemet 100 and Madopar 125 containing smaller amounts of levodopa allow a more accurate titration of the dose. Before the introduction of dopa-decarboxylase inhibitors the commonest limiting factor to the use of levodopa was gastro-intestinal upset with nausea and vomiting. Now it is psychiatric. Patients who cannot take levodopa find that even in small doses it makes them uncontrollably agitated or gives them hallucinations. Simple overdosage produces facial twitching. In spite of these disadvantages levodopa has made the life of the Parkinsonian patient much more bearable. When levodopa does not work amantidine 100 milligrams twice daily can be tried or any of the older anticholinergic drugs such as benzhexol (Artane) 5 milligrams, or orphenadrine (Disipal) 50 milligrams, both taken three times a day.

RESPIRATORY SYSTEM

Age brings with it a gradual decline in pulmonary function and an increased tendency to respiratory infections. Pneumonia is a common terminal event and most of the old people who come to necropsy show evidence of it even when they have also had some other serious disease such as cancer or a stroke. A common dilemma, when an old person gets pneumonia, is when to regard it as "the old man's friend" and when as a disease demanding urgent treatment. If it has been possible to get a complete picture of the patient with a fractured femur it is also usually possible to determine in which patients the fracture is itself part of the terminal illness. For such patients antibiotic treatment may be withheld if there is no hope of obtaining any beneficial result. Pneumonia is not always a consequence of the fracture, and, it may have been the cause. It is well established that old people may suffer what have been called premonitory falls at the onset of any acute illness but especially pneumonia. Pneumonia is also a hazard if the fall causes not only a fractured femur but a fractured rib.

Bronchitis is common in old age, particularly in old people who smoke. Chronic bronchitis in the elderly has its ups and downs as it does in younger patients but it is rare for it to present with extreme respiratory failure as is seen in middle age. It is always worth estimating the degree of airway obstruction and the Wright Peak Flow Meter is a useful piece of equipment in any geriatric ward. Patients with bronchitis demand antibiotic treatment as long as the sputum is purulent and the general condition improves if this is done. There seems little to choose between the broad spectrum antibiotics for old people with bronchitis; amoxycillin, tetracycline, cephalexin and cotrimoxazole are equally effective.

Because of the anoxaemia they cause, both pneumonia and bronchitis are liable to precipitate heart failure with or without arrhythmias and the patient may need a diuretic as well as an antibiotic. Digoxin will be needed when there is atrial fibrillation. Pulmonary complications after operation are more likely to occur if the patient continues to smoke up to the time of operation. The patient with a fractured neck of femur has no choice but, for elective surgery, even a week's abstinence from smoking will be well repaid in the period after operation.

ANAEMIA

A fractured femur causes acute bleeding and requires a transfusion of two or three units of blood. This makes it hard to estimate the incidence of anaemia. It is known that one in three of old people admitted to hospital have haemoglobin levels of less than 12 grams per 100 millilitres. Of these two thirds have iron deficiency anaemia, often associated with gastro-intestinal blood loss from hiatus hernia, peptic ulcer, diverticular disease, haemorrhoids or cancer of the gastro-intestinal tract. Drugs causing gastro-intestinal blood loss, for example aspirin, phenylbutazone and other antirheumatic drugs, are likely to be the cause of anaemia in patients with arthritis.

A substantial minority of anaemias are due to deficiency of vitamin B_{12} or folic acid. Such patients show a macrocytic picture, megaloblastic change in the marrow and low levels of one or both haematinic factors in the blood. A patient's vitamin B_{12} status is accurately reflected by the serum level but folic acid is better estimated in the red cells rather than the serum. Megaloblastic anaemia, particularly when due to deficiency of folic acid, may be associated with mental confusion. Provided the diagnosis is correct, megaloblastic anaemias respond very well to treatment.

Normocytic anaemias are common in patients with chronic sepsis, especially if there is a pressure sore, an abscess or a sinus. They are also seen in patients who are chronically ill with malignant disease, renal failure or rheumatoid arthritis. They do not normally respond well to iron. The patient often needs transfusion unless the cause can be eliminated. Mild degrees of anaemia do not greatly increase the surgical risks, but they may delay recovery and rehabilitation after operation. The haemoglobin should, therefore, be estimated before the operation and regularly afterwards.

ALIMENTARY SYSTEM

Apart from constipation, which is nearly universal, disorders of the alimentary tract do not play a large part in the wide spectrum of diseases seen in the elderly orthopaedic patient. Hiatus hernia, peptic ulcer and diverticular disease are mainly important as sources of anaemia due to occult bleeding. Hiatus hernia is a common cause of vomiting and sometimes of haematemesis in geriatric wards. It usually responds to simple medication with alkalis, perhaps best if combined with alginates as in Gaviscon. Diverticular disease is a common cause of abdominal pain and disturbed bowel function in the elderly. It is best treated with bran, preferably given as the natural substance. If this is unacceptable the patient may take it as a prepared breakfast food or as a high fibre crispbread.

Rectal examination is an essential part of the assessment of the patient and is normally undertaken as part of the examination of the abdomen. The principal value in the orthopaedic patient is in the exclusion of faecal retention. In men it enables the prostate to be felt. In women it may reveal a pelvic mass. In both sexes the state of the anal sphincter is important. Rectal prolapse will not be detected unless a rectal examination is done.

GENITO-URINARY SYSTEM

Renal function falls by half between the ages of 20 and 80. Many elderly people get on well with blood urea levels between 8 and 16 millimols per litre (50 to 100 milligrams per 100 millilitres) but their reserves are slender and they are easily tipped into serious renal failure by conditions which reduce glomerular filtration. Chief of these is dehydration which accompanies any condition impairing the patient's ability or willingness to drink. Dehydration is aggravated by fever, vomiting and diarrhoea. Reduced cardiac output as in cardiac infarction, heart failure or shock, all common hazards which may accompany a fractured femur, have the same effect. Renal failure may also result from severe urinary infection and urinary retention. The latter is suggested by the finding of a distended bladder which may be entirely asymptomatic. None of these factors, dehydration, impaired cardiac output, retention of urine and infection are mutually exclusive and all may be present in one patient. They justify the routine examination of blood urea levels in every old person who is admitted to hospital. Although in theory the estimation of the serum creatinine level should be more accurate we have not found it helpful.

Examination of the urine is relatively unhelpful in the elderly. Most specimens contain a small amount of protein which is of little significance. The test for sugar is often unreliable because old people commonly have a high renal threshold for glucose. It is very difficult without catheterisation to obtain reliable specimens from old people for microscopy and culture. Midstream specimens are something of a lottery. Routine cultures of midstream urine specimens show that as many as half of the elderly women in hospital have a urinary tract infection. Most are asymptomatic and do not need any treatment. Indeed, culture of control catheter specimens show that almost half the positive results in mid stream specimens are due to contamination. If antibiotics are given they relapse soon afterwards. We no longer use antibiotics unless the patient has symptoms such as frequency, dysuria, recent incontinence, confusion, fever or general malaise. Urinary infections are not always benign, however, and deaths from renal failure do occasionally occur.

Urinary retention is quite a common problem after orthopaedic operations as it is in the elderly generally. In men it is usually due to prostatic hypertrophy and requires a consultation with the urologist. In women the cause may be faecal impaction, stroke or the so called atonic bladder. In both sexes retention may be precipitated by over enthusiastic fluid intake, a brisk diuresis or the use of atropine like drugs which affect the function of the bladder. These include the tricyclic antidepressants and the anti-cholinergic drugs used in the treatment of Parkinsonism. Men with retention require to be seen by the urologist but women may respond if the offending drug is removed and any faecal impaction dealt with. Those who do not will require to be catheterised for a time until the bladder regains its tone. It is customary in such patients to introduce a catheter for one week. This is then removed to see whether bladder function has returned. If it has not the patient is catheterised for a further week, and this regime continued for as long as necessary. Most patients recover in a few weeks.

MALIGNANT DISEASE

Every series of old people with fractures contains patients with malignant disease and myelomatosis. Sometimes they have sustained a pathological fracture. Sometimes they have had an ordinary traumatic fracture and the cancer is an incidental finding. At Hastings about one patient a month with malignant disease is admitted to the orthopaedic department with a femoral neck fracture. When there is any doubt in the surgeon's mind a biopsy is taken at the time of operation.

Myelomatosis may be recognised by the finding of a paraprotein on electrophoresis of the serum and by the presence of anaemia. Cytotoxic agents such as cyclophosphamide and melphalan often produce worthwhile prolongation of life.

EYES AND EARS

Poor sight and hearing both make their own contributions to the risk of accident and cut patients off from the community. About 20% of our patients with fractured femora have defective eyesight and most of them are already known to the Eye Department. It is important, however, not to overlook any steps which may improve the patient's sight and hearing. A simple ear trumpet made from a plastic funnel and a length of plastic tubing is a valuable piece of ward equipment. It is important also to make sure that a patient's hearing aid, if she has one, is in working order. Her spectacles also should be checked.

DRUGS

An important element in the medical assessment of an old person at any time is to consider her drugs. Old people metabolise drugs less efficiently and excrete them more slowly than do the young. At the same time because of the increased incidence of illness in old age and the problems of multiple pathology, they are more likely than the young to receive medication, often for more than one disease. Indeed, the side effects of one drug may be taken as an indication to prescribe yet another.

All this increases the possibility of drug interaction with unfortunate side effects. The list of drug interactions grows every year. It involves particularly those drugs which are bound to proteins such as anticoagulants, aspirin, phenylbutazone and chlorpropamide. Interaction may also involve drugs which are metabolised in the liver such as vitamin D and barbiturates. Antibiotics such as tetracycline may not be absorbed if the patient is taking iron. Diuretic therapy leads to potassium loss and sometimes therefore to increased sensitivity to digitalis. Drug interactions apart, simple over prescribing is always a hazard. There is a tendency, when any medication is prescribed to relieve some distressing symptom, for the patient to believe that he must take it for the rest of his life. Many tranquillisers, sleeping tablets, diuretics, drugs for the relief of rheumatic pain, and even digoxin are taken in this way. Thus, every time the patient develops a new symptom, she acquires another drug on permanent prescription.

Antihypertensive drugs are important in improving the life expectation of younger patients but there is little evidence that they do good in the elderly. They are far more likely to upset old people by their side effects, causing postural hypotension with faintness, dizziness and a tendency to fall. Sleeping tablets, tranquillisers and antidepressants also cause faintness due to postural hypotension and may themselves be the cause of falls and fractures. To simplify a patient's drug regime is often an easy way to improve her wellbeing.

Terminal Care

About 20% of patients referred to the geriatric orthopaedic unit after being operated on for femoral neck fractures die within two months of operation. This is quite a high mortality but perhaps not surprising when one takes into account the high incidence of concomitant disease and the fact that the average age of the patients is over 80. This mortality is certainly acceptable when one considers the alternative to operation in a patient with a fractured femur, the bedfast state with continued pain and difficulty in nursing.

Many of the patients who do not long survive their operation succumb to pneumonia, stroke, cardiac infarction or occasionally pulmonary embolism. A minority of patients, however, follow a prolonged downhill course, perhaps with pressure sores. It is essential that the patient's progress is reviewed regularly and that futile and perhaps inhumane attempts at rehabilitation are abandoned when there is little prospect of recovery. This, however, must be a positive decision by the medical staff in consultation with the other members of the team, particularly the nurses. Once a decision has been made that the team is conducting terminal care and not rehabilitation, a new set of priorities come into existence. It remains necessary to review the patient's progress on every ward round with as much care as before; it is essential to make sure that the patient is free of pain; and finally that she has every opportunity to unburden herself of her anxieties.

Further Reading

Aaron, J. E., Gallacher, J. C., Anderson, L., Stasaiak, L., Longton, E. B., Nordin, B. E. C. and Nicholson, M. (1974). Frequency of osteomalacia and osteoporosis in fractures of the proximal femur. *Lancet* **1,** 229-233.

Agate, John (1970). "The Practice of Geriatrics", 2nd Edn, Heinemann, London.

Beals, R. K. (1972). Survival after hip fracture. *Journal of Chronic Diseases* **25,** 239-245.

Brocklehurst, J. C. (1977). "Textbook of Geriatric Medicine and Gerontology", 2nd Edn, Churchill Livingstone, London.

Campbell, A. J. (1976). Femoral neck fractures in elderly women. *Age and Ageing* **5,** 102.

Clarke, A. N. G. (1968). Factors in the fracture of the female femur. *Gerontologia Clinica* **10,** 257-270.

Dequeker, J. (1975). Bone and Ageing. *Annals of the Rheumatic Diseases* **34,** 100-115.

Exton Smith, A. N. (1973). Osteoporosis. *Nutrition (London)* **27,** 116-125.

Hodkinson, H. M. (1975). "An Outline of Geriatrics". Academic Press, London.

Irvine, R. E., Bagnall, M. K. and Smith, B. J. (1977). "The Older Patient", 3rd Edn, English Universities Press, London.

Isaacs, B., Livingstone, M. and Neville, Y. (1972). "Survival of the Unfittest". Routledge, Kegan Paul, London.

Jenkins, D. H. R., Roberts, J. G., Webster, D. and Williams, E. O. (1973). Osteomalacia in patients with fractures of the femoral neck. *Journal of Bone and Joint Surgery* **55B,** 575-580.

Kanis, J. A., Fitzpatrick, K. and Strong, J. A. (1975). Treatment of Paget's Disease of Bone with Porcine Calcitonin. *Quarterly Journal of Medicine (N.S.)* **44,** 399-413.

Medicine in Old Age (1974). *British Medical Journal,* London.

Nicolaides, A. N. (1975). "Thrombo embolism". Medical and Technical Publishing Co., Lancaster.

Norton, D., McLaren, R. and Exton Smith, A. N. (1975). "An Investigation of Geriatric Nursing Problems In Hospital", 2nd Edn, Churchill Livingstone, London.

Pitt, Brice (1974). "Psychogeriatrics: an introduction to the psychiatry of old age". Churchill Livingstone, London.

3

Anaesthesia in the Elderly

A. M. HAINES

Introduction

When the age of the population served by a hospital is so high that about half the patients on an ordinary orthopaedic operation list are geriatric, then the experience of anaesthetising such people over the years gives confidence in their management so that, except for certain definite indications, all elderly patients will be accepted for operation under general anaesthesia.

Before operation a careful history, examination and preparation are as important as the anaesthetic itself because, in the operation theatre, the patient will have the absolute attention of the anaesthetist with controlled ventilation of the respiratory system and monitoring of the cardio-vascular system if required. Thus, nowhere will a geriatric patient be safer than during this time.

It is most important to have a close liaison with the medical, surgical and geriatric disciplines, so that the patients are in the best possible physical condition before operation and also so that all treatment is fully co-ordinated. Emergency resuscitation has its own very definite principles which are dealt with in Chapter 4.

Management Before Operation

For an elective operation the ideal is to have every patient seen in an anaesthetic clinic a short while before admission. There a careful history will allow assessment of the previous health of the patient and will give certain guidelines in the clinical examination.

For the patient admitted as an emergency, such as a fracture near the hip, the same principles will apply and as many preparatory investigations should be done as is possible without unduly delaying the operation. A radiograph of the lung fields is a necessity as is often an electrocardiograph. Any abnormality found needs intensive measures to rectify it; for example, a pleural effusion found and aspirated need not postpone the operation unless the underlying cause is itself a contra-indication. A cardiac abnormality, such as an undiagnosed auricular fibrillation may need to be controlled by appropriate measures, but the importance of the operation to the wellbeing of the patient may outweigh the desirability of a long course of medical treatment; the latter often being more beneficial after a painful orthopaedic lesion has been dealt with.

Haematological studies are done routinely, including the serum electrolytes, potassium, sodium and blood urea. An alteration from the normal may indicate that there has been malnutrition, dehydration or potassium loss from the prolonged use of diuretics. Many old people who look after themselves at home have neither an adequate diet nor take regularly the drugs that have been prescribed because of decrepitude preventing proper preparation of food, forgetfulness or mild dementia preventing a normal daily routine and even financial problems causing embarrassment in shopping. Drugs cause a special problem; often so many are prescribed that the elderly patient becomes muddled and may take one drug but not the other, such as the diuretic drug but not the potassium supplement.

Anaemia must be corrected by giving oral or intravenous iron. When time is insufficient blood transfusion may be necessary but this is not the ideal method because it is easy to overload the circulation. Blood transfusion just before operation on an old person with anaemia is especially bad, because, if the venous return to the heart is poor, the transfusion increases the venous engorgement and as a consequence increases the risk of local venous congestion and congestive heart failure.

It is important to consider all drugs that must be continued, particular emphasis being placed on those taken for diabetes, cardiac conditions and rheumatoid arthritis.

Physiotherapy will be directed towards proper breathing exercises and postural drainage of the chest and must be intensive if there is any evidence of bronchitis or if other causes of mucopus are found. Smoking should be stopped, if possible, for at the least one week before admission.

CARE OF THE SKIN

Good nursing ensures that the patient comes to the operation theatre as mentally and physically fit as possible and in particular the care of the skin must be maintained while the patient is on the theatre table by the careful positioning of pads and rubber mats to prevent undue pressure. Even one hour of excess pressure on the heel or the sacrum can dispose to a bedsore in a weak and anaesthetised patient.

PREPARATION

As is usual, anaesthesia is divided into preparation, premedication, anaesthesia during operation and, last, the time of recovery. The choice of anaesthetic will vary, not only with each anaesthetist, but also with each patient and each operation.

More care than usual must be taken to ensure that the elderly patient, often frightened and a little confused, takes no fluid or food by mouth four hours before induction of anaesthesia because of the usual dangers of inhalation of stomach contents. This needs very careful nursing attention because of the inability of some geriatric patients to appreciate instructions and the willingness of a neighbouring patient to give misguided assistance.

Premedication should start on admission to hospital if the patient is very nervous, and in any case on the night before the proposed operation to ensure a good night's sleep with freedom from pain. Barbiturates must be avoided in the elderly because of the confusion that can be caused by such drugs. Nitrazepam 2.5 to 10 milligrams (Mogadon) or diazepam 2 to 10 milligrams (Valium) therefore are commonly used as night sedatives. Many patients have their own specific drug which may be continued for the time being and later changed if it is not a satisfactory regime. The analgesics useful in the elderly and which do not cause too many side effects are soluble aspirin and codeine compound, dextropropoxyphene and paracetamol (Distalgesic) and pethidine. Papaveretum 10 milligrams and soluble aspirin 500 milligrams in an effervescent base is a particularly good preparation for elderly patients with severe pain from orthopaedic conditions.

The time during the day at which the operation will be done must alter the medication given; if the operation is to be towards evening the nervous patient will be kept calm by giving diazepam 5 to 10 milligrams either by mouth or by intramuscular injection on the morning of the operation. There should never be an artificial ruling of nothing to eat or drink on the day of operation; old people do not take well to such abstinence, but must only be starved for the four hours or so before the operation.

PREMEDICATION

Premedication is given about one to one and a half hours before the anaesthetic.

There are many useful combinations but two or three that have been found very valuable are, first, pethidine 100 milligrams, perphenazine 5 milligrams and atropine 0.5 milligrams and, finally, phenopiridine 1.0 milligram and droperidol 1.0 milligram. Each combines a sedative with an antisialogogue. Should the patient have a contra-indication to a sedative then atropine 0.5 milligrams alone is satisfactory.   The doses given above are an average and every patient must be assessed by weight, general condition and, particularly important, by age, which necessitates a reduction in the dosage, before the drugs are prescribed.

Perphenazine has been found to be most useful in certain conditions. When given with pethidine it produces good sedation with little dis-orientation, it is a good antisialogogue and it helps to relax the smooth muscle of the bronchi if there is spasm. Atropine is also useful for its antisialogogue action and although it does cause some stimulation of the central nervous system this is not a problem when used in ordinary doses. Again it must be emphasised that every patient is dosed according to the condition and in the very old the dose can be reduced to half or less of that which is necessary for a fit young adult.

The patient who has much bronchospasm is best treated by aminophylline 360 milligrams given the night before operation as a suppository and repeated with the premedication. This will facilitate ventilation and expectoration and will allow better aspiration of mucopus from the lungs during, and at the end of, anaesthesia than would otherwise be the case. Although the drug can give rise to tachycardia it is not dangerous, provided this is recognised; then the anaesthetist will not have anxiety and give unnecessary medication to control the heart rate.

Hydrocortisone 100 milligrams must be given by intramuscular injection to any patient who has had prolonged treatment with corticosteroids during the last 12 months and who may have an impaired response to stress because of a depressed suprarenal function. Without the availability of the estimation of routine blood corticol levels, reliance must be placed on the clinical signs, notably changes in the blood pressure and the pulse rate unrelated to other causes, in deciding if more hydrocortisone is needed during and after the operation. It is possible that hydrocortisone predisposes to an increased rate of venous thrombosis and delay in wound healing, and although this has not been found noticeable in Hastings the dose is kept as low as possible.

THE ANAESTHETIC

The three phases of anaesthesia, induction, maintenance and recovery are well recognised, but to the geriatric patient it is the latter that needs the greatest care because the patient is no longer under the immediate control of the anaesthetist. Blocking of the airway can easily develop by lying the patient in an incorrect position, with the jaw and tongue falling or secretions pooling in the pharynx. Even a short period of hypoxia can cause hypotension with subsequent cerebral damage and perhaps death. Therefore all such patients must be nursed in a recovery area with a well qualified nurse in constant attendance and who, under no circumstances, will leave her patients until recovery is so far advanced that it is safe for transfer back to the ward. If recovery is not satisfactory no chances should be taken but the patient kept in the intensive care unit until the condition is normal.

Induction
For the induction there are the usual drugs, such as sodium thiopentone 2.5%; methohexitone 1%; Althesin; nitrous oxide and oxygen; cyclopropane and oxygen, and others.

The choice of any particular agent to be used is not only the personal choice of the anaesthetist, but also that dictated by the needs of the patient. The length and severity of the operation and the time to recovery afterwards are important. Particularly must the elderly patient being dealt with as a "day case" be given a suitable anaesthetic to allow quick recovery. The general condition of the patient will influence the choice; for example, the avoidance of thiopentone in ill patients, particularly those with fixed cardiac output, or those in shock. Such patients have little response to the fall in blood pressure which may occur after the administration of this drug. The other intravenous agents, methohexitone and Althesin also need the same care as sodium thiopentone. For the elderly out-patient Althesin is a satisfactory choice if an intravenous induction agent is needed because it is eliminated more quickly than are barbiturates; there is, however, no advantage in its use for in-patient anaesthesia because of the short time over which it acts. Therefore methohexitone is used for routine operations. Althesin must be avoided if there is bronchospasm which may be exacerbated. For the patient who is very frail a nitrous oxide to oxygen 70% to 30% mixture followed by the addition of a volatile agent such as halothane gives a very satisfactory induction.

The dose of any drug used in induction is that which is necessary to produce sleep. When it is necessary to anaesthetise a patient who is in a state of shock and who has peripheral vasoconstriction a most useful agent is cyclopropane in 50% mixture with oxygen because such patients do not tolerate induction by intravenous drugs well. After induction it is desirable to intubate all patients (with the exception of the shortest procedures) with a cuffed oral endotrachial tube of the largest size that will not damage the trachea or larynx. This is facilitated by the use of 50 to 100 milligrams of succinyl choline intravenously as soon as the patient is asleep; after ventilating the patient three or four times with oxygen the tube is passed. Regurgitation at this stage can be dangerous unless equipment for suction of the pharynx is readily to hand; a further precaution is to give gentle cricoid pressure during the intubation. Geriatric patients do not seem to develop the muscle pain which often follows the use of succinyl choline in fit young people, but care must be taken to see that the paralysis has worn off before repeating the dose or using another relaxant. This precaution must be taken to avoid any chance of confusing the action of different drugs at the end of the operation when the patient is to start normal breathing.

Maintenance of Anaesthesia
The choice of whether to retain natural respiration or to paralyse the patient and control the ventilation depends on the operation to be done. If it is small and a tourniquet is to be used then all that is really necessary is adequate analgesia. Such patients should be allowed to maintain normal respiration after intubation using a mixture of nitrous oxide with 30% oxygen with the

addition of a volatile agent such as halothane in its lowest concentration possible. To avoid liver damage no patient exposed to halothane should receive it again within three weeks, within which time either methoxyflurone or trichlorethylene can be used.

Should the patient, because of a necessary position on the table, or by the nature of the operation, be subjected in any way to the slightest possibility of being unable to maintain an adequate ventilation of a total volume of nine to ten litres a minute, controlled respiration must be used. A long acting muscle relaxant, such as d-tubocurarine, gallamine or pancuronium are given followed by intermittent positive pressure ventilation. Adequate analgesia must be maintained and intravenous pethidine in 25 milligram doses but not more than 100 milligrams in any two hours, fentanyl in 0.05 milligram doses or halothane, methoxyflurone or trichlorethylene are satisfactory for this purpose. Careful observation of the colour, skin temperature and sweating of the patient, and the associated rise in pulse and blood pressure when painful stimuli occur will indicate the need for additional analgesia.

Induced hypotension
There need be no hesitation in lowering the blood pressure in a geriatric patient when indicated, provided that the proper precautions are taken and that its problems are well understood (Grace, 1961). Much more often than not the hypotension will so shorten the time of operation that it is beneficial to the patient as well as the surgeon. For certain procedures such as spinal decompression for paraplegia caused by metastases it is essential. Further, by reducing blood loss to one quarter of what it might have been without hypotension the progress after operation will be better because large transfusions of blood will not be needed.

The contra-indications to hypotension are coronary ischaemia, cerebro-vascular disease or any severe coexistent disease causing great debility.

Hypotension is produced by combining reduction of cardiac output with ganglion blockade and the use of posture to help gravity to empty the circulatory system in that part being operated upon.

Ventilation is controlled at a rate of seven to ten litres a minute with nitrous oxide 70% and oxygen 30%. Halothane, in a concentration sufficient to produce a fall in the systolic blood pressure to 80 millimetres of mercury is added. Should this, together with intermittent positive pressure ventilation not give a satisfactory fall of pressure in five to ten minutes, a ganglion blocking agent such as pentolinium 2.5 to 5 milligrams (Ansolysin) as an initial dose is given, starting with a small dose as it is potentiated by the other agents. Vasodilation can be started with the patient horizontal and then posture can be used to increase the fall in blood pressure and venous drainage at the operation site. Occasionally, should a tachycardia develop, it may be necessary to give a beta blocker to slow the heart rate. Practolol is one of the drugs of choice.

Great care must be taken in the earlier stages of the anaesthetic to see that induction is smooth, that no coughing occurs and that there is no cyanosis, all of which increase venous congestion and so obviate the effects of the hypotension produced. Always there must be continuous monitoring of the blood pressure.

During the operation fluid loss must be replaced. At first about 1 litre of Hartmann's solution should be given to cover the withholding of fluid before operation; after this blood should be given to keep pace with the loss, which must always be measured by weighing the swabs.

When the end of the operation is approaching the muscle relaxant is reversed by the intravenous injection of atropine 1 milligram followed by neostigmine 2.5 to 5 milligrams and normal respiration is encouraged.

After hypotension it is particularly necessary to monitor the blood pressure carefully in the stage of recovery. This must continue not only until the patient has regained vasomotor control, but until that control is stable. A head down tilt should be maintained until the effect of the ganglion blocking agent has worn off—a good indication of the latter being the return of the normal size of the pupils and their reaction to light. Should the patient for some reason have to be put into the head up position the legs must be raised to prevent pooling of blood in them.

In order to try to prevent deep venous thrombosis and consequent pulmonary emboli certain precautions are taken. Macrodex may be given during the operation and thereafter one bottle each day for three days in an attempt to prevent sludging of the platelets. On the operation table the calves of the patient should neither be left hanging over the end of the table at any time, nor should they rest flat during long procedures, when the heels should be padded and raised to hold the legs off the table.

Calcium heparin 5000 International Units subcutaneously may be given 12 hourly to those patients in whom the risk of thrombosis and pulmonary emboli are known to be considerable, but this will increase the blood loss after operation.

Recovery

At the end of the operation the patient is positioned on the side if this is surgically practical and then placed on a tipping trolley which must carry oxygen. On the way to the recovery area a trained nurse will always walk beside the head of the patient so that she may watch the airway carefully and give oxygen immediately if it is necessary.

In the recovery area the patient is monitored for pulse, blood pressure and respiration. Suction and oxygen are available for every patient.

It is at this time that the patient is most at risk and needs to be watched and nursed by highly skilled staff. There is always danger of a sudden fall in blood pressure, regurgitation and inhalation of stomach contents or obstruction of the airway which can pass almost unnoticed if attention is diverted elsewhere; this can so easily occur if the patient is being nursed in an ordinary but busy ward. The anaesthetist must be told of any untoward change found by monitoring.

When a patient is considered safe and fit to be moved, return to the ward is arranged. The time spent in the recovery area will vary with the age, general condition and rate of recovery of each individual, but at least four hours must pass after the use of ganglion blocking drugs before sitting up is allowed.

Pain relief after operation is very important in an old patient and must be done with great care so that there is freedom of movement in bed and also to give confidence to the patient who will usually be out of bed and walking the next day. After certain operations such as total hip replacement the surgical relief of pain is good and only one or two doses of opiates may be needed. Thereafter an excellent analgesic is papaveretum 10 milligrams and soluble aspirin 500 milligrams taken together, with nitrazepam added at night if necessary. Excessive complaint of pain must never be ignored because often it is an indication of some surgical complication and should be investigated fully.

Nausea and vomiting after operation needs the exhibition of perpenazine (Fentazin) 5 milligrams twice a day by injection. The dose should not exceed this because although it is a very valuable drug it can give rise to side effects in the extrapyramidal system, occasionally with occulomotor crises. If Fentazin does not control the symptoms metoclopramide monohydrochloride (Maxolon) 10 milligrams can be given three times a day; extrapyramidal tract side effects are found much less often with this drug, although they can still occur.

A haemoglobin estimation is made 48 hours after a major operation to help decide if the patient needs further blood transfusion.

Early mobilisation together with the routine use of antibiotics in orthopaedic patients greatly help to lower the number of chest complications after operation. Also the policy of operating on all fractures in the elderly within 24 hours of admission instead of some days later allows the patients to be up again before broncho-pneumonia has occurred. Good medical care, light anaesthesia, short operating time with the least possible blood loss all contribute to the success of surgery in the aged and maintain a low morbidity and mortality.

References

Grace, A. (1961). Prostatectomy under hypertensive anaesthesia. *Proceedings of the Royal Society of Medicine* **54,** No. 12.

4

Resuscitation in Geriatric Orthopaedics

H. MIDDLETON

Geriatric orthopaedic patients can present either as an emergency after an accident or by elective admission for the treatment of progressive joint disease or some similar disabling condition. Many of the latter patients will need replacement arthroplasty. In this chapter the resuscitation problems of the patient admitted in either situation will be considered.

The availability of an operating session every day of the week has been an important factor in influencing the methods used to resuscitate the geriatric orthopaedic patients at Hastings. It is possible to obtain the best conditions for surgery with neither undue haste nor excessive delay. The nurses on the wards, the operation theatre staff and the supporting services are available without the need for the attendance of on-call personnel at night. The normal practice is, therefore, to operate on emergency patients within 24 hours of admission.

Complications Before Operation

The hazards complicating emergency surgery can be formidable but the difficulties can be overcome or mitigated. Practically none of our patients has been refused operation because of being unfit for anaesthesia; such a refusal is almost inevitably followed by death. Energetic resuscitation and the proper surgery at the right time will, at the least, make the patient free of pain and at best, able to return home. Nevertheless we "do not strive officiously to keep alive" patients in whom death appears inevitable.

Elderly patients, when admitted as an emergency, have many other conditions, some of which may be contributory factors to the injury. Pneumonia or arteriosclerotic heart disease may confine the patient to bed from which they may fall on attempting to get up for any purpose. Little strokes or mental impairment can cause a careless attitude to danger, falls in the home or road traffic accidents. Diabetes may have been unsuspected or may be uncontrolled and must always be looked for very carefully in such patients.

Many of the conditions in the elderly may not have been diagnosed nor treated before admission but many others, both real and imaginary, will have been treated by a multiplicity of medicines, of which many are self-prescribed. Persistent questioning of the elderly and those close to them is usually rewarded by a collection of drugs which have not been mentioned because they were not thought to be relevant to orthopaedic surgery. Some, such as corticosteroids, are of great importance in resuscitation. Elderly patients with aches and pains often take aspirin in its various forms. The blood examination may reveal hypochromic anaemia and the stool may be positive for occult blood.

BLOOD TRANSFUSION

The resuscitation of most emergency geriatric orthopaedic patients demands the transfusion of blood both for the correction of known or suspected anaemia or hypovolaemia and for the replacement of blood sequestered at fracture sites and associated contusions. Very large amounts of blood are thus lost; Fuchsig *et al.* (1967) quantified blood loss in surgery of the hip and showed that as much as 2.5 litres might be lost in the first three days. The correction of this loss is therefore of primary importance. Because most of our patients are operated upon within 24 hours it is seldom necessary to start blood transfusion before operation and it is an advantage to set up the drip after the anaesthetic has been induced. The patient is asked before-hand whether he is right or left handed and the dominant side is not chosen for the drip. Once anaesthesia is established the resultant vasodilatation allows the insertion of a large plastic cannula (14 Gauge) and a long central venous pressure catheter without distressing the patient. The anaesthetist is able to secure temporary access to a smaller vein with a scalp vein needle. The importance of placing an efficient drip should not be underrated. At any time subsequently it may become necessary to transfuse a large amount quickly. The skin is cleansed with an organic iodine preparation. The cannula is handled with aseptic precautions and, once in position and the drip running well, it is firmly fixed with adhesive plaster and plaster of Paris bandage as well if there is any possibility of lack of co-operation and interference after operation. Splinting of the elbow is avoided.

Under anaesthesia, vasodilatation and the large cannula greatly assist the rapid transfusion of blood. Packed cells are particularly useful for the correction of pre-existing anaemia and substantially reduce the risk of overload. Packed cells are preferred to whole blood in acid citrate dextrose (A.C.D.) solution. Whole blood is diluted 25% by A.C.D. and the red cells lose their ability to survive at about 1% a day from the time of donation. Whole blood in A.C.D. near the expiry date is worth only about 50% of the value of the blood it replaces. This must be taken into consideration in deciding how much blood is to be given and at what rate. It may be necessary to attempt to obtain fresher blood. Additional blood may be necessary a few days after the transfusion of long dated blood. Calcium gluconate, 10 millilitres of a 10% solution is always given after each litre of whole blood.

TOURNIQUETS
When operations are done under tourniquet the hyperaemia which occurs when the pressure is released may be massive and may lead to sudden central hypovolaemia and hypotension. Two tourniquets should never be released simultaneously. Adoption of the head-low position is usually sufficient to maintain control. Oxygen is given and the vital signs are observed most carefully until stability returns.

HYPOTHERMIA
This is a common finding in the elderly in Great Britain. Fox *et al.* (1973), found 10% of a group of 1000 to have a deep body temperature below 35.5 degrees Celsius in an English winter of January to March 1972. Severe hypothermia, well below 35 degrees Celsius (95 degrees Fahrenheit) has been present in some of our patients with fractures who have lain unable to summon help and inadequately clothed until discovered some while later. It is essential that the body core temperature be raised rapidly to allow surgery to be done. The common method is to immerse the torso in warm water but this is not acceptable in the presence of severe injuries. Intermittent positive pressure ventilation (I.P.P.V.) with oxygen is used. The inspired gases are passed through a heated humidifier and delivered to the endotracheal tube at a temperature of 40 degrees Celsius. The torso only is warmed by water tube blankets or by a heating cradle. Subsequent heat loss is reduced by wrapping the patient in aluminium kitchen foil or a "space blanket".

Arterial samples are taken for blood gases and pH at frequent intervals until the arterial oxygen improves to near normal (95 to 100 millimetres of mercury) and until the combination of the administration of 8.4% sodium bicarbonate intravenously and artificial ventilation with a high minute volume has brought the pH within normal limits (7.35 to 7.42). This may take some hours while normal circulation returns to the periphery. All fluids given intravenously are warmed by passage through a warming coil and the rate and quantity given are adjusted according to the central venous pressure (C.V.P.) levels. Ledingham and Mone (1972) recommended that the aim should be a rise in temperature of 0.5 to 1 degree Celsius per hour.

When the temperature measured by a thermistor probe in the oesophagus or the external auditory meatus reaches 35 degrees Celsius active rewarming ceases to avoid an excessive after-rise.

DEHYDRATION
Dehydration is often found in patients admitted in emergency. Intravenous

fluids are given as the treatment of first choice. Oral fluids need to be withheld a few hours before operation to avoid a full stomach. The use of an ultrasonic nebuliser to produce a fog of water or saline for the patient to breathe is advantageous because it prevents the normal fluid loss at expiration and may, perhaps, allow an intake. Also it reduces latent heat loss and it prevents mucus from thickening, thus assisting expectoration and preventing the formation of mucus crusts. A nebuliser may be used in conjunction with an oxygen mask of the Venturi type, the fog being offered to the air entrainment ports.

CORTICOSTEROIDS

These are no substitute for blood, fluids, electrolytes and oxygen but once these latter have been attended to corticosteroids are a most useful adjunct and our attitude to them has been liberal. Fractures are a severe stress to the elderly and at least 200 milligrams of hydrocortisone (Efcortesol) or 4 milligrams of dexamethasone (Decadron) are given intravenously if a low blood pressure persists. No axiomatic figure for a low blood pressure can be given because so many of the elderly will have been hypertensive before the injury. An intelligent assessment based upon the feel of the radial artery and the appearance of the fundi may be the best that can be done.

The corticosteroids may be repeated, such as hydrocortisone 100 to 500 milligrams three or four times in 24 hours or dexamethasone up to 80 milligrams a day. Severe shock may require a bolus intravenous dose of 2 to 6 milligrams of dexamethasone (Decadron) per kilogram of estimated body weight to be given and repeated, if necessary, in two to six hours.

ELECTIVE SURGERY

Patients awaiting elective surgery should be as fit as possible and certain important measures should be taken before admission to reduce to the least possible the chance of a collapse that will lead to the necessity of resuscitation. The time a patient spends on the waiting list will vary; but his condition may differ markedly from that when first seen to that at the time of admission.

At the anaesthetic clinic an appraisal and assessment of the risks are made and methods decided upon in order to promote the best conditions for the patient at, and after, the operation to avoid the necessity of resuscitation.

Anaemia down to 10 grams per 100 millilitres may be corrected by iron, folic acid and cyanocobalamin (Vitamin B_{12}). Below that level, or if there is shortness of breath at rest, blood transfusion of packed cells is given on admission. Iron dextran infusion (Imferon) is contra-indicated in rheumatoid conditions. Weight reduction has often been ordered in the treatment of orthopaedic complaints but dietary restraint is best discarded in the last few days before admission to prevent the liver from being inadequately protected.

The respiratory peak flow is measured at the clinic because it is a useful indicator of difficulties that may present at or after operation. Improved respiratory performance may be obtained by physiotherapy, bronchodilators, antibiotics or chemotherapeutic agents. Sometimes it is advisable to plan the operation on a patient with severe chronic bronchitis to take place in the summer months. A peak flow of less than 250 litres is a warning that particular attention must be given to oxygenation after the operation.

Patients with heart disease will have an electrocardiogram before operation which is to be kept for reference purposes. If the condition is one that it is possible to improve the patient is referred to a cardiologist for treatment; many drugs, such as the beta blockers, practolol (Eraldin), propranolol (Inderal), oxprenolol (Trasicor) may be prescribed, as may a digitalis preparation such as digoxin (Lanoxin) or a diuretic such as frusemide (Lasix. These drugs may need to be altered or withdrawn before, during or after surgery. The cephalosporin antibiotics often used in geriatric orthopaedics as a cover for joint replacement may become more nephrotoxic in the presence of frusemide which is, therefore, stopped while cephaloridine or cephalexin (Ceporin or Ceporex) is being given. If beta blockers are continued during operation, atropine is given in high dosage (1 to 2 milligrams intravenously) to protect against vagal dominance.

Patients suffering from osteoarthritis can be expected to sustain considerable blood loss at or after arthroplasty when much work has had to be done on the bone adjacent to the joint because of the proliferation of blood vessels in this condition (Trueta and Harrison, 1953). Replacement of this loss must be allowed for in planning transfusion needs.

General Principles of Resuscitation

OXYGEN

The basis of resuscitation lies in ensuring that the blood is well oxygenated and circulating properly. The blood requirement has been considered above. Oxygen is much simpler to obtain and to administer than blood and it is usually very difficult to find any reason for withholding it. Oxygen may be needed at any time for the treatment of circulatory collapse with hypovolaemia or hypotension or in those patients admitted to hospital suffering from a concomitant pneumonia, hypothermia or the respiratory depressant effect of narcotics. A high concentration, such as 60%, is used in the short term while the underlying problem is identified and treated. One of the various transparent plastic masks which covers the mouth and nose is adequate if the patient is breathing spontaneously. Nasal catheters are useful if the patient is breathing through the nose but care must be taken to make sure that the catheters do not advance too far because the gas can then expand the stomach which may cause the diaphragm to splint the lungs or worse still, cause regurgitation of stomach contents leading to asphyxia or Mendelson's syndrome (Mendelson, 1946).

Breathing is like justice, not only must it be done, it must be seen to be done. To maintain the warmth of geriatric patients by covering them up to an extent that prevents movements of breathing being seen properly is a temptation which must be resisted. If the respiration is shallow, when the tidal volume will probably be low, a mechanical or manual ventilator is used until the cause has been identified and corrected. Possible causes include sudden changes of posture in bed or on transfer between departments and iatrogenic conditions such as nitrous oxide asphyxia, caused by the anaesthetic gas being released from the blood to the lungs, or residual curarisation if a muscle relaxant used during the operation has not been properly metabolised or antagonised. Cyanosis persisting in spite of assisted ventilation and in the presence of apparently adequate lung expansion must be attributed to cardiac causes, fat embolism, thrombo-embolism or pulmonary micro-embolism. These latter must be treated urgently and energetically but the outlook is poor in this age group.

After operation oxygen is given even when the breathing appears adequate. There is almost certainly a degree of intra-pulmonary shunting, some of the blood passing through airless or collapsed alveoli and returning to the circulation unoxidised. Oxygen masks giving a constant fixed percentage of oxygen in air entrained into a Venturi chamber (Ventimasks) are used. These deliver at 24, 28 and 35% of oxygen identified by one, two or three rings on the body of the chamber. Hypoxaemia may cause the patient to become confused or restless. It is important not to give narcotics in the belief that pain is the cause until the oxygenation has been checked. A fatal respiratory depression could result.

THE PLACE OF PHYSIOTHERAPY

Physiotherapy to the chest is made difficult by the presence of untreated fractures but after the operation the pain caused by movement should have been in great part alleviated. After consciousness has returned postural drainage, assisted coughing and thoracic vibration may be used. Inhalation of nebulised sterile saline loosens secretions and promotes expectoration; doxapram hydrochloride (Dopram) is given intravenously if it is necessary to stimulate deep respiration.

In the supine position the dependent bronchi fail to drain. The resultant atelectasis causes shunting and hypoxaemia particularly in the paravertebral areas. As soon as is possible the patient is turned to either side or placed prone or sitting up at suitable intervals and within the limits set by the surgical condition. Each position should be held long enough for adequate drainage and coughing. To facilitate the toilet of the upper respiratory tract in the very frail patient a tongue suture is sometimes valuable. A mono-filament suture is passed from side to side through the tongue towards its base; the knot is tied well outside the mouth. This suture is removed as soon as the patient no longer needs assistance with expectoration.

PAIN RELIEF DURING RESUSCITATION

The elderly patient with fractures may have severe pain, shock and hypoxaemia. Strong analgesic drugs are needed but they should be given well diluted and intravenously; titration by the doctor over a period of 20 to 30 minutes until a satisfactory level of analgesia is achieved is the best method. Morphine or pethidine have been our choice on most occasions. If the intravenous route cannot be used, and it must not be used if the patient is not fully observed, then the deep intramuscular route of the lateral thigh is chosen. Quite apart from the danger of injection into the sciatic nerve there is never justification in rolling a patient with fractures to inject into the buttock. "Little and often" is the analgesia regime of choice.

An infusion of ethyl alcohol 5% in saline or dextrose may provide a useful euphoria in those accustomed to its use. It is in addition a valuable source of calories.

Notable relief from pain occurs when fractures have been fixed and the dosage of the drugs being used then needs to be reviewed.

Vasopressors are seldom indicated, most episodes of hypotension responding to the infusion of blood or dextran of 70 000 molecular weight (Lomodex 70 or Macrodex) or to the intravenous corticosteroids. If these measures are insufficient metaraminol bitartrate (Aramine) is the drug most likely to be useful. It is given as an infusion containing 15 to 100 milligrams (1.5 to 10 millilitres) in 500 millilitres of isotonic saline or 5% dextrose and no other dilutent should be used. A response may be expected within two minutes and the rate of infusion is adjusted to maintain the desired level of blood pressure once this has been reached.

TREATMENT OF CARDIAC ARREST

Cardiac arrest occurring in the operating theatre is treated by the medical team already present. Arrest elsewhere is dealt with by a "mayday" call through a radio paging system which summons medical staff and the equipment for inflation, intubation, defribillation, monitoring and the administration of certain drugs at any time of the day or night. Any member of the hospital staff can call "mayday" if a patient seems to be in trouble. The senior person on the spot is the one who decides to start cardio-pulmonary resuscitation (C.P.R.). The decision to stop C.P.R. and to accept that death has occurred is taken by a doctor. This may not be very difficult in some of the very severe risk emergencies. It is less simple when the patient has been admitted for elective surgery and had a reasonable expectation of life. Tracheal intubation gives the best and most effective inflation of the lungs. Even in experienced hands a mask is seldom a good fit on an aged, edentulous face.

Closed chest cardiac massage is performed while the patient is artificially ventilated. Fractures of the ribs are frequently reported in the elderly subjected to C.P.R. but all staff are assured, both in lectures and at the incident, that fractures are an accepted complication and that they must not feel that they have done anything wrong should this happen.

The appearance of the pupils is none too useful a guide to the success or otherwise of C.P.R. in the elderly (Gilson 1965) and reliance should not be placed on this sign.

The presence of a femoral pulse shows that compression of the heart is effective. The electrocardiogram is placed in position once C.P.R. is in progress. Countershock is applied via external electrodes if ventricular fibrillation is present.

Sodium bicarbonate 8.4% is always given intravenously to correct metabolic acidosis no matter how short the arrest. Various other drugs such as lignocaine, (Xylocard 2% bolus injection), calcium chloride or adrenaline may be required.

If C.P.R. is effective and a spontaneous heart beat returns the patient is transferred to the intensive care unit and monitored continuously until recovery is deemed complete. Artificial ventilation continues for a long time after the return of the heart beat.

No individual doctor or nurse is expected to remember all the steps of C.P.R., the controls of the equipment, the drugs, where to find them and how much to give. Every ward and every department has a complete set of instructions on all these matters spread out on a large board which can be taken to the patient.

Parameters and Charts

The time of skilled nurses is too valuable to be wasted on unnecessary charting. The protocol should demand the useful minimum of records to be kept and as the patient progresses measurements may be recorded at less frequent intervals until abandoned altogether. There are many occasions on which measurements such as blood pressure are made every few minutes but charted only when some significant change occurs or at fixed intervals much longer apart.

TEMPERATURE

Hypothermia in the elderly is a possibility never to be overlooked even in the most unlikely circumstances. Temperature is measured on admission, on return from surgery and at predetermined intervals. These intervals are short if there are departures from acceptable limits.

Hypothermia developing before admission or during operation, or from the transfusion of cold blood or intravenous fluids, may render the patient unresponsive to resuscitation until the temperature returns near to normal. Shivering makes very heavy demands on metabolism and should not be permitted. It may be prevented by intravenous chlorpromazine (Largactil) given slowly in dilute solution intravenously until the shivering ceases.

BLOOD PRESSURE

Readings are frequent, perhaps at ten minute intervals if it seems low for the individual. This is continued until the patient has made an adequate response to treatment. Any fall in the systolic pressure of 25% or so is a cause for concern. It may be the first sign of infarction either myocardial or pulmonary in the elderly in whom pain or respiratory distress may be absent or unremarkable. All falls in blood pressure require that the wound dressings and closed drainage be inspected.

CENTRAL VENOUS PRESSURE

This is a useful parameter in that the manometer is constantly visible. Provided there is a rise and fall with respiration, being evidence that the catheter is patent, the height is a good guide to the administration of blood or other intravenous fluids. Should the level fall below 6 centimetres there may be vasodilatation or hypovolaemia and the drip rate of infusion may have to be increased: above 16 centimetres there may be overtransfusion and the need for a vasodilator drug or digitalis. Ten to 12 centimetres of the fluid in use is the level usually aimed at, that is, 20 to 22 centimetres above the imaginary hard surface upon which the patient lies.

PULSE

This is best observed continuously on a simple electronic display and rate meter. It is charted every 15 minutes during the first few hours after the initial resuscitation, after the operation or after a "mayday" call.

ELECTROCARDIOGRAPH

Irregularities in the electrocardiograph are fairly common in the elderly and a tracing before the operation is obtained for comparison in the event that any change should occur after operation. If there is any cause for concern the electrocardiograph is displayed on an oscilloscope. Adherent terminals on the chest are preferred to avoid constricting bands on the limbs.

RESPIRATION

Any upward trend in the rate usually indicates atelectasis. If it does not revert after a change in posture and encouragement to expectorate the physiotherapist is called to assist the coughing up of the plug of mucus which is almost certainly the cause of the trouble. Further active intervention may be required such as catheter suction or bronchoscopy if physiotherapy does not produce relief. An antibiotic should be used thereafter.

FLUID CHARTS

The 24 hour clock is used and the charts are balanced at midnight. Each fresh chart must detail the fluid intake for the next 24 hours; this will be amended in the light of new biochemical or haematological data as well as being related to the fluid output. The elderly are normally intolerant of too rapid transfusion and it is important to give one twenty-fourth part of the day's fluid in each hour. Special transfusion sets which have a second calibrated chamber to simplify this regime are available (Soluset 100, Abbott). Successful measurement of the urinary output requires the use of an indwelling catheter. This will also simplify the observation of glycosuria of which there is a high random incidence in the elderly.

Most facets of resuscitation can be predicted, all can be prepared for and none must come as a surprise.

References

Fox, R. H., Woodward, P. M., Exton-Smith, A. N., Green, M. F., Donnison, D. V. and Wicks, M. H. (1973). Body temperatures in the elderly, a national study of physiological, social and environmental conditions. *British Medical Journal* **1,** 200.

Fuchsig, P., Brücke, P., Blumel, G. and Gottlob, R. (1967). A new clinical and experimental concept on fat embolism. *New England Journal of Medicine* **276,** 1192.

Gilson, A. (1965). Clinical and biochemical aspects of cardiac resuscitation. *Lancet* **2,** 1039.

Ledingham, L. McA., Mone, J. G. (1972). Treatment after exposure to cold (letter). *Lancet* **2,** 534.

Mendelson, C. L. (1946). Aspiration of stomach contents into lungs during obstetric anaesthesia. *American Journal of Obstetrics and Gynaecology* **52,** 181.

Trueta, J., Harrison, M. H. M. (1953). Normal vascular anatomy of femoral head in adult man. *Journal of Bone and Joint Surgery* **35B,** 442.

5

Diabetes and the Geriatric Orthopaedic Patient

HAROLD BRODRIBB

The hospitals in Hastings serve an unusually elderly population and each year there are about 200 new patients in the diabetic clinic; most of them are over 50 and many over 65 years of age. Also the clinic, which stands at 1200 attendances has a net gain of 50 to 60 new patients every year.

Elderly diabetic patients are very liable to the complications of their disease such as peripheral neuropathy, ischaemia and sepsis from any trivial lesion; further, impaired vision leads to bruises and falls and all of these may call for orthopaedic advice.

There are, less often, occasions where the instability of the diabetes leads to an orthopaedic disaster. For example, a keen lady gardener on insulin, and forgetful of meals, tended to become hypoglycaemic. Aged 72, she fell, suffering a compound fracture of the tibia and fibula, on which she tried to walk. Later this came to amputation. Four years later, again in hypo-glycaemia, she fell and fractured the shaft of her femur. Happily, treatment was successful and she attended the clinic, walking with the aid of one stick only, until she died aged 87.

What standard of care is necessary for the elderly diabetic? All are agreed that no standard is too high for the younger patient; but there are some that consider that dietary restrictions and routine urine tests are a needless burden on the elderly. Ultimately complications may be inevitable with advancing age and duration of diabetes; but experience has led to the conviction that it is the poorly controlled diabetic who suffers earlier and more severe complications. The most careless diabetic, observed here since childhood, had had a stroke, was partially blind and had died of uraemia before he was 40 years old.

In the elderly it is right to aim at normoglycaemia throughout most of the day. Because a high proportion develop a rising renal threshold, blood glucose estimations should, ideally, be observed at each attendance. Although it may not be possible to achieve this in a provincial centre with, perhaps, an overworked laboratory, nevertheless the attempt should be made. The patients' own urine tests must, however, be repeated in the clinic at each visit. If this standard of care is not maintained, the condition of any diabetic suddenly faced with a surgical emergency is all the more hazardous and the operation may have to be delayed.

The essential purpose of follow-up care in a diabetic clinic is preventative, with the avoidance if possible of complications, both orthopaedic and general, as well as maintenance of good diabetic control.

The conditions most frequently calling for collaboration between the departments are the diabetic foot and lower limb, the treatment of fractures and, finally the elective treatment of arthrosis.

The Diabetic Foot

This condition was well described by Oakley et al. (1956) and by Catterall (1972). The careful assessment of the varying factors of neuropathy, ischaemia and infection is essential as a guide to successful treatment.

NEUROPATHY

There is progressive loss of pain, temperature appreciation, vibration sense and ankle reflex. Examples, not uncommon, serve best to depict the dangers of this condition. Thus, an elderly man was admitted with extensive scalds on the lower back and abdomen. He had been unaware that he was taking too hot a bath until he sat down. Again, a woman developed a dangerously ischaemic foot, after buying shoes much too small, because they were in a sale. No normal person could have stood the very acute discomfort that was caused. Insensitive corns, callosities and deformed toenails are especially dangerous and, without the invaluable help of highly trained chiropodists, many disasters would occur.

ISCHAEMIA

The foot is cold—often palpably—as compared to the other. The peripheral arteries, and sometimes the popliteal and femoral arteries, are only felt with difficulty or not at all.

The skin at first is pale and waxy with loss of hair. The refilling of capillaries after pressure is slow. Intermittent claudication may be admitted on enquiry, but sometimes it is the skin circulation only that is impaired. Ultimately the foot, or limb, has a dusky appearance and rest pain occurs, the leg often being hung out of bed at night. By this time, any demand for additional blood such as is caused by infection, a friction sore or burns, will be the last straw and gangrene will ensue.

SEPSIS

Acute

Corns, callosities and deformed toenails have been mentioned, but any skin lesion, such as tinea or eczema, often provides the portal of entry. Rarely, the infection may be very acute, with severe cellulitis, high fever or even septicaemia. Identification of the organism and correct antibiotic treatment is urgent and the cure can be dramatic. The condition may lapse into a chronic state requiring months of bed rest and perhaps operation.

Chronic

Some patients, with a slightly impaired circulation, have such severe sensory loss that they do not seek advice until the lesion has advanced considerably. Many diabetic patients, including some of those newly referred, may have walked for many weeks on a huge, necrotic and all but painless ulcer. The immediate treatment is radical removal of all dead or dying tissue to allow free drainage of the depth of the ulcer. A swab is taken to identify the organism, and for a guide as to the correct antibiotic treatment. If there is the slightest surrounding cellulitis systemic antibiotics may produce a dramatic improvement and, despite not knowing the organism, a broad spectrum antibiotic (such as Magnapen) should be given forthwith.

Dry gangrene, or a dry scab on a healing lesion calls for antibiotic powder. But any moisture, especially below a hard slough, needs the careful removal of the latter followed by the application of Aserbine cream or continuous eusol dressings.

It is surprising how much excavation can be done quite painlessly in the diabetic clinic, including the removal of nails and large callosities. Great care must be taken with septic blisters, which must always have a swab taken for culture. In diabetic patients infections may come to the surface some distance from the deeper primary lesion. The whole track must be carefully opened up to allow free drainage at the source. A radiograph of the area for bone infection must complete the investigation.

The chronic indolent ulcer is disheartening to both patient and doctor. The variety of dressings used confirm this, ranging from antibiotic creams to eusol, Aserbine, honey, insulin, cod liver oil and red lotion. A possible vitamin C deficiency must not be forgotten. Sometimes zinc sulphate, 220 milligrammes three times daily by mouth, improves the speed of granulation and epithelialisation, and should be given a trial in case there is zinc deficiency, but after months of care many such patients still come to operation.

Fractures in Diabetics

Impaired peripheral and proprioceptive sensation and defective vision all predispose to falls.

The commonest fracture is of the neck of the femur, which, in common with other less disabling fractures, will inevitably exacerbate the diabetic state, depending on the degree of shock and lack of accustomed activity and an increase in the antidiabetic drugs is nearly always needed.

Pain, distress, anxiety, sudden immobility and increased suprarenal activity all raise the blood sugar level; occasionally this may not occur if the degree of shock is sufficient to have caused suprarenal exhaustion.

This is why the physician must treat each case individually and not by any standard routine. An instant blood sugar estimation must be taken on admission and repeated later. Without this repeated and carefully assessed investigation hyperglycaemia will certainly occur and, when it does, it must be noted that it may be the first warning of the onset of infection in any part of the body such as in the lungs or in the genito-urinary tract, especially after catheterisation.

Elective Operations

Corrective operations for arthritis often need special care by the physician, especially the rheumatoid patients who may have been or who are still on steroid treatment which may have originally precipitated the diabetes. Variation of the dose of steroids will be an extra factor, requiring special vigilance around the time of operation.

MEDICAL CARE AT THE TIME OF OPERATION

Because, at Hastings all the acute surgery is done in a hospital three miles from that which contains the medical wards, there are no junior medical staff available so it has to be the senior staff who are called up for advice in an emergency.*

It is of the greatest importance that all diabetic patients facing an operation which may occasion their biggest diabetic crisis should have the highest calibre of advice and the personal supervision of a physician fully conversant with the treatment of diabetes.

It is essential to have an immediate estimation of the blood sugar, followed by three hourly urine tests, and further blood sugars, if the first is much abnormal. These must be done in the laboratory for the best results, but if the tests cannot be done quickly, then the bedside use of Dextrostix or of the Ames reflectance meter, are useful substitutes but accuracy will vary with the experience of the user. The former is more accurate at the lower blood sugar levels, and is valuable in detecting hypoglycaemia. The latter is needed to determine high levels of blood sugar. The laboratory estimation is always to be preferred, and, in the case of the severely ill patient, must be done, and insisted upon, whatever the hour.

*This is in great part why no diabetic patient is delayed to any extent before an emergency operation and also why these patients run an almost normal course thereafter. (Editor)

TREATMENT BEFORE OPERATION

Each patient presents an individual problem. The aim must be to achieve a blood sugar at the time of operation near the top limit of normal, that is, approximately 150 to 200 milligrammes per 100 millilitres.

Emergency cases

Patients on diet and oral treatment   These can usually be controlled on diet alone. The blood sugar may be hardly disturbed but, if it is raised, the necessity for speed may justify a small dose of soluble insulin, such as 6 or 10 units. The fast before the anaesthetic is often sufficient to restore a normal blood sugar, which should be estimated again at the time of anaesthesia.

A large number of older patients are on oral treatment. At Hastings, most are on chlorpropamide, between 100 and 400 milligrammes once a day, but a few have, in addition, a slow release capsule of phenformin S.R. 50 milligrammes once or—rarely—twice a day. The long action of these drugs must never be forgotten, and, if the emergency has caused an unusual fast, hypoglycaemia must be excluded. If confirmed, it needs instant treatment by glucose, preferably intravenously, giving 25 millilitres of 25% solution, especially if an operation is imminent. This dose may have to be repeated before or during operation.

Patients on insulin or diagnosed as diabetic on admission   These present the most urgent problem. The former may be hypoglycaemic, if meals have been omitted, but this could be offset by the emotion and pain of the accident, and the blood sugar can remain high. This will invariably be the case if all insulin has mistakenly been omitted and also in the diabetic newly discovered on admission. If operation is to be undertaken speedily, urgent action is essential to obtain frequent urine observations and blood sugar estimations to enable the correct insulin needs to be determined. When the usual daily dose of insulin is known, this will also help in estimating the initial dose of soluble insulin, and the size of doses at subsequent intervals. The effect of any dose of a long acting insulin given before admission must not be forgotten. The dose of soluble insulin is always related to, and judged by, the blood sugar level and also by the circumstances of each patient. If given six hourly, one should rarely recommend more than 20 units at each dose and often it can be smaller. Only rarely, such as in a precomatose condition with acidosis, is a larger dose required. In these cases, with a very high blood sugar, one or more four hourly doses may be needed to achieve a blood sugar level at which an operation can be safely performed. An intravenous glucose infusion is better given at this stage even if more insulin is needed, in order to avoid ketosis. To decide on the type of infusion the electrolytes must also be estimated, especially the potassium, because its level can fall dangerously if the blood glucose has been lowered quickly.

Elective cases

It is highly desirable for the physician to have adequate warning not only of the operation but also of the time at which it will be done. A fast of up to six hours before the anaesthetic must be planned and related to the diabetic treatment.

Those on diet and oral treatment   Well controlled patients on diet alone, or on small doses of oral drugs, merely omit food and drugs on the morning of operation. If it is to take place in the afternoon they may have up to 15 grammes of carbohydrate in a drink, on waking, the blood glucose usually remaining controlled by the oral treatment of the previous day.

Those patients who are on large oral doses will have a similar preparation for a morning operation but they may need a small dose of insulin later in the day, on recovery from the operation. If the latter is late in the day, they may receive half their normal oral dose with the morning carbohydrate drink. If the urine or blood sugar levels are low at midday, an intravenous dose of 25 millilitres of 25% glucose is then necessary.

It is helpful if all diabetics are admitted at least 24 hours before operation.

Patients on insulin   For these patients it is essential that they be admitted at least one full day ahead of operation. Many patients are on long acting insulins, or a mixture of them with soluble insulin given each morning. In all but the most trivial operations, the insulin must be changed temporarily to the soluble variety given 12 hourly. If these patients are not already well controlled a small booster dose up to 10 units of soluble insulin at midday or at midnight may also be needed.

About three quarters of the normal requirement of insulin is given at 8 a.m. and if the operation is in the morning, intravenous glucose, 25 millilitres of 25% is given instead of breakfast. This is repeated according to the urine or blood sugar, at midmorning or on the operation table.

If the operation is in the afternoon, glucose or other carbohydrate drinks can be given up to six hours before the anaesthetic, and subsequent meals replaced by intravenous glucose as described above. Frequent urine, and occasional blood sugar, tests before operation are advisable. If the results are higher than expected the intravenous glucose is omitted.

Treatment at and after Operation

During operation the main diabetic risk is hypoglycaemia. If this is suspected, a blood glucose, if only by Dextrostix, must be done at once. However, adherence to the regime described above rarely makes this necessary.

The behaviour of the blood glucose after operation always presents an individual problem, and varies with the patient and what has been done.

Ideally a blood glucose should be estimated within two or three hours, and is essential if no urine is obtainable. Otherwise two or three hourly urine tests must be observed. This should be done hourly when a catheter has been left in place.

The physician must follow these results, and not act on any rigid pattern. Experience shows that there is always some reaction after operation, which varies individually and which will be accompanied by a lowering of the blood sugar during shock after which it will then rapidly rise as the patient recovers. The evening dose of soluble insulin, if it is normally needed, must be delayed until the first evidence of a rising blood glucose is obtained. A small increase in glycosuria is sufficient evidence. This is the time for a small dose, perhaps half the usual one, of soluble insulin, and, if that has been underestimated in this reactionary phase, a further dose must be given six hours later. The nature of any intravenous infusion must be considered, and it is much easier if this contains glucose all the time, rather than if this is suddenly cut off by changing to normal saline. Electrolytes also require assessment.

It is important to get back as soon as possible to 12 hourly soluble insulin—morning and evening—but if perchance that dosage has been underestimated it should be followed by small midday and midnight booster doses of 10 units, if glycosuria reaches 2% or higher, and 6 units for three quarter per cent or 1% respectively at the midday or the midnight tests. The actual dose of these six hourly boosters can safely be added to the preceding main dose on the following day, that is, 10 units required at midday can be added to the dose at eight o'clock the next morning, and the same procedure followed by the addition of midnight boosters to the dose at six o'clock the next day. In this way the need for these midday and midnight boosters will usually be cut off quickly and automatically. If complications occur extra doses may be needed for some days, even if they cause a considerable rise in the morning and evening main doses. This is the most rapid way of stabilising the patient, and more efficient than the usual method of using a "sliding scale".

At this stage many new factors must be observed and anticipated. Fever, pain and urinary, chest or wound infection may cause a large increase in insulin requirements. Such a need is often the first indication that all is not well. Conversely, decrease of pain or anxiety, a drop in fever, and increasing mobility, all demand a drop in insulin. Food intake at this time may also be varying. Constant adjustments of dose must be anticipated during the convalescent period, and if possible the patient must be restored to the usual type and routine of insulin or oral treatment before going home; should this not be possible before discharge, the normal routine is to be restored as soon as possible under out-patient supervision. All patients should go home with instructions to expect a cautious reduction of the requirements for diabetic control as the general condition returns to normal. The patients, or the District Sister, must constantly watch the urine tests and, for the first few days at home, it is wise to do them more often than twice a day to get an early warning of the need for adjustments of dosage.

The art of stabilising an elderly diabetic is largely one of intelligent anticipation, and an attempt must always be made to try to teach the patients to do this themselves. Further, it is the role of the physician to keep his geriatric diabetic patients as fit as possible all the time, to teach them how to look after themselves and to take over their care immediately in any crisis, whether it be orthopaedic or otherwise, so that the surgeon can proceed at once to operate on a diabetically fit patient.

Advances in the treatment and management of diabetes proceed apace; this chapter has given the methods practised over many years. Recent advances just being incorporated, such as the Ames reflectance meter which has become more readily available for in-patients and out-patients, now makes it easy to have frequent and accurate blood sugar estimations. Further, new types of insulin are being introduced and other oral drugs are replacing chlorpropamide. Phenformin is also being replaced at many centres. The treatment of diabetic coma, or incipient coma, is greatly improved by the use of continuous intravenous insulin. Nevertheless, it is the need for individual control by an experienced endocrinologist that remains essential to prevent the various crises and complications of diabetes that occur in the geriatric patient.

References

Catterall, R. C. F. (1972). *British Journal of Hospital Medicine* **7**, 224.
Oakley, W., Catterall, R. C. F. and Mencer Martin, M. (1956). *British Medical Journal* **2**, 953.

6

Rheumatoid Arthritis in the Elderly

IVAN WILLIAMS

Rheumatoid arthritis is a chronic inflammatory disease usually affecting multiple joints, occasionally limited to a few, but rarely monarticular. Apart from obvious involvement of joint and periarticular structures, other systems may be involved. Therefore eye, skin, renal, cardiovascular, respiratory and alimentary lesions are not uncommon. Haematological abnormalities are the rule in both established and in most of the early cases.

Unfortunately, the aetiology of the disease remains as obscure in the elderly as in the young. For some years auto-immune reactions have been considered to play a fundamental causative role, mainly because of the biochemical changes found in rheumatoid sera and because of similarities between rheumatoid arthritis and other diseases such as Hashimoto's thyroiditis and systemic lupus erythematosis, in which autoantibodies frequently occur. So far, however, there is no evidence to suggest that these reactions are primary factors rather than secondary manifestations to other stimuli such as infection, hypersensitivity or injury.

Organisms of the Mycoplasma and Diphtheroid groups have been recovered from synovial membrane and fluid from joints affected by rheumatoid arthritis and from tissue culture preparations of rheumatoid synovial fluid (Bartholomew, 1965; Duthie *et al.,* 1967). It has been suggested that patients with this disease have abnormal immune responses to commonly encountered organisms. This abnormal immune response may itself be the result of metabolic deficiencies. Suffice to record that so far no convincing evidence has come to light to substantiate this theory although recent work on viruses and arthritis appears promising.

Of all other suggested aetiological factors ranging from psychological to dietary factors, heredity receives substantial support from many surveys (Empire Rheumatism Council 1950; De Blécourt *et al.,* 1961; Lawrence and Ball, 1958). Clinical, radiological and serological evidence of rheumatoid arthritis appears to be four times as frequent in families with positive sheep cell tests. The test itself is positive in three times as many relatives of rheumatoid arthritic patients as in controls (Ziff *et al.*, 1958). Therefore, there appears to be sufficient evidence to conclude that there is a familial incidence of rheumatoid arthritis although genetic transmission has not been proved (Blumberg, 1960).

Although the cause is unknown, statistics relating to the prevalence, age at onset and sex ratio have been fairly accurately evaluated.

In the United Kingdom it is estimated that 1% of the male and 3% of the female population suffer from rheumatoid arthritis in one form or another. The mean age of onset is in the early part of the fourth decade but there appears to be a marked increase in women affected between the ages of 50 to 55 (Empire Rheumatism Council, 1950; Short *et al.*, 1957). The incidence is also apparently higher in the underprivileged social classes.

From these figures it is obvious that most patients with rheumatoid arthritis in the geriatric population will be widows, probably in economic distress, posing severe social as well as medical problems. Most of such patients rely on social security for adequate aid; on the voluntary "meals on wheels" service for an occasional hot midday meal, if such a service exists, its absence being only too frequent in rural areas.

For a widow with disabled hands, cooking may become difficult and even dangerous and increasing reliance will be placed on easily prepared and often cold meals. The basis of such meals will be bread and tea—the geriatric "haute cuisine". It is no surprise to find only too often that the elderly rheumatoid woman is thin.

Impairment of mobility and the general lack of home help facilities makes housework difficult.

So, with the inexorable contracture of the environmental perimeters, these patients become hostages to their disease, living in squalor, underfed, frequently socially forgotten, stripped of human dignity until they are admitted to a geriatric bed or sink in solitude into their lonely graves.

The pathology of the disease may vary in severity from joint to joint in the same patient. The articular changes begin in the synovial membrane which proliferates, becomes hyperaemic, villous and infiltrated with inflammatory cells. Synovial fluid increases; it becomes less viscous and cellular and contains enzymes which may damage cartilage. Granulation tissue spreads from the periphery and destroys cartilage and produces subchondral erosions.

Later, capsular, tendon and muscle damage occurs with adhesion formation and contractures. This process may cease spontaneously at any stage and of course can be modified by active treatment.

The extra-articular pathology can embrace all systems producing sub-cutaneous nodules, pleuritic and parenchymatous lung lesions; and arteritis which may secondarily affect renal function or produce the symptoms of polyneuritis and myositis which often play an unrecognised part in aggravating the patient's physical disability.

Median or lateral tarsal nerve compression are often unrecognised complications leading to intrinsic muscle weakness in the hands and feet—such weakness can aggravate dysfunction already existing in these muscles and which is recognised as being such an important factor in the production of deformity.

Necropsy findings show evidence of pericarditis in a significant number of patients who had rheumatoid disease—in many cases unsuspected during life. Histological examination of the bundle of His may reveal rheumatoid nodules explaining the not infrequent conduction defects seen on the electrocardiograph.

Sjögren's syndrome can be distressing to an elderly patient who may already have some loss of smell or taste.

Mild eye complications may similarly aggravate pre-existing visual difficulties and, although fortunately rare, severe eye complications unless energetically treated may rob the patient of sight.

To expect to identify all such pathology as part of the rheumatoid process in a geriatric patient would be optimistic. Most people reach old age through minefields of illhealth, and frequently bear the scars of earlier skirmishes with disease and perhaps deprivation. In addition, the inexorable progress of tissue degeneration, particularly that affecting the locomotor system, makes accurate differentiation between similar pathological appearances and lesions caused by dissimilar agents almost impossible.

The presenting symptoms of rheumatoid disease are similar in the elderly and the young. The onset is frequently acute and rapidly progressive; occasionally the disease may be monarticular or affect few joints but a polyarthritis is most commonly seen. The cardinal symptoms of morning stiffness, joint pain and tenderness, fatigue and general malaise, coupled with the signs of hot, swollen joints, tendon and muscle weakness, restricted joint movement, contractures, impaired mobility and function, with perhaps nodule formation, arteritic and neuritic changes indicating systemic involvement are seen at all ages.

However, the elderly, in contrast to the young and middle aged, are invariably scarred by degenerative changes or previous illness which produce confusing physical signs and complicate interpretation of radiological, haematological and biochemical findings.

In less acute cases the onset of definite joint symptoms may be preceded by malaise, fatigue, loss of weight and perhaps indications of peripheral nerve compression such as carpal tunnel syndrome.

Unexplained oedema of the lower legs, ankles and feet may be attributed falsely to cardiac or renal disease whereas the true cause may be in the adjacent joints.

Erosive changes in the cervical spine do produce neurological signs common to other degenerative conditions; muscle wasting, a normal accompaniment of ageing, can progress rapidly and become irreversible if aggravated by further neuritic and articular insults.

The immobility and loss of independence commonly affecting the elderly rheumatoid patient is frequently due to neurological and muscular deficit rather than articular inflammation.

Differential Diagnosis

Degenerative joint disease, either primary or secondary, is obviously the most important condition when considering the differential diagnosis. Primary osteoarthrosis is universal in the elderly and may produce severe pain, particularly in weightbearing joints, of which the hips and knees are those most frequently affected. However, the first carpo-metacarpal joint is frequently affected in women and, perhaps, in common with Heberden's and Bouchard's Nodes, often lead to an erroneous diagnosis of rheumatoid disease.

In general, the monarticular onset of degenerative joint disease is gradual and although the affected joint may be swollen it seldom shows the synovial proliferation seen in rheumatoid arthritis. Tendons are rarely affected and systemic involvement does not occur. In primary osteoarthritis the radiological changes of osteophytes, sclerosis and loss of joint space contrast with the erosive changes and periarticular osteoporosis of rheumatoid arthritis, which also produces disastrous joint derangement and deformity which is rare in osteoarthritis; however, weak intrinsic muscles of the hand can produce moderate ulnar deformity and even subluxation in the elderly without there being either an underlying inflammatory or degenerative arthritis present.

Degenerative joint disease can produce severe pain but the ill, careworn appearance common in rheumatoid disease is rarely seen in the absence of an inflammatory arthropathy.

Haematological and biochemical investigations do not have the same specific diagnostic importance in the elderly since abnormalities may be multifactoral in origin. Nevertheless, primary osteoarthritis in the healthy is not usually associated with high erythrocyte sedimentation rate, a low haemoglobin or positive tests for the rheumatoid factor.

The so called mixed arthritis, generally accepted as degenerative joint changes superimposed on rheumatoid arthritis or other inflammatory joint disease—or vice versa—can produce diagnostic problems. If the inflammatory arthropathy preceded the degenerative changes, then a carefully taken history will usually reveal the fact, although it must be remembered that rheumatoid disease rarely becomes inactive.

When a low grade rheumatoid arthritis is superimposed on osteoarthritis then diagnosis can be difficult, particularly where weightbearing joints are involved. When there is doubt it is probably safest to assume the condition to be rheumatoid disease until proved otherwise.

Psoriatic arthritis may be indistinguishable from rheumatoid arthritis but usually there are clinical differences. The disease is less severe, running a more remitting course and not infrequently involving the terminal inter-phalangeal joints and sacro-iliac joints only, an unusual feature in rheumatoid disease. Although the arthritis may precede the skin lesions, it is rare for this to happen in the elderly. However, the psoriasis may not be widespread and careful examination of the nails and scalp is important when the condition is suspected. Occasionally, a severe destructive type occurs, producing terrible deformities of the hands (the so called arthritis mutilans). Most patients are sero-negative for the rheumatoid factor but it is not unusual to find slightly elevated serum uric acid levels because of increased nucleic acid turnover in the skin lesions (Steinberg et al., 1951; Bermann and Jillson, 1961; Bremner, 1966).

Primary gout becomes clinically more frequent as age increases. In the early episodic stages the diagnosis is usually relatively easy. If, however, the chronic stage has been reached unrecognised, with an active polyarthritis, joint damage and deformity, then the diagnosis may be difficult. In the elderly, hyperuricaemia may be secondary to factors other than gout, for example renal insufficiency or diuretics (Lewis, 1961). In such cases a search for urate crystals in synovial fluid, and histological examination of possible tophaceous material may be needed to establish the diagnosis. Radiological evidence in most patients is inconclusive and the erythrocyte sedimentation rate, not surprisingly, may be raised since there is often considerable synovial inflammation.

The test for the rheumatoid factor is usually negative but because rheumatoid arthritis and hyperuricaemia can co-exist the possibility of the former must be considered seriously. When in doubt a diagnosis of rheuma-toid arthritis should be assumed until proved otherwise because this disease is more likely to cause rapid and severe joint damage.

Suppurative arthritis, although uncommon, is seen more frequently in the elderly, particularly affecting joints already damaged by pre-existing arthritis. Although a joint infection is usually accompanied by severe pain, swelling and systemic involvement, the presence of chronic active rheumatoid disease may mask the infection and the symptoms be attributed to a local exacerba-tion of the disease. Unless the joint is aspirated and the synovial fluid cultured the true nature of the illness may be missed, leading to a fatal bacteraemia.

An infected joint may masquerade as an acute exacerbation of a generalised arthropathy or the systemic manifestations may be obscured by chronic illhealth. Although rheumatoid disease may present in an acute monarticular form, the possibility of a single infected joint must always be considered. The only infallible method of establishing the diagnosis is by aspiration and culture; microscopy and cell counts are rarely conclusive because synovial fluid from a swollen rheumatoid joint may be very cellular and contain "pus" cells.

Polyarthritis not uncommonly accompanies or precedes the appearance of neoplastic disease. In particular, neoplasms of the bronchus or pleura may be associated with severe joint pain and swelling, to the extent that the condition is indistinguishable from rheumatoid arthritis. Remission often occurs if the neoplasm is removed, treated with cytotoxic drugs or radiotherapy (Williams, 1960). For this reason full clinical examination and chest radiography are mandatory for patients presenting with an arthropathy, particularly when there is unexplained systemic involvement.

Polymyalgia is a common locomotor disease of patients over 60 (Dixon *et al.*. 1966), particularly affecting women. The distribution of shoulder and pelvic girdle stiffness and pain without peripheral joint involvement is usually sufficient to make a clinical diagnosis. However in mild affections the possibility of rheumatoid arthritis cannot be always excluded; further confusion can be caused by the presence of a raised erythrocyte sedimentation rate, abnormal globulins and perhaps a positive test for the rheumatoid factor. In contrast to rheumatoid disease and despite the severe incapacity and pain most patients appear and feel well. Very rarely polymyalgia may progress to a generalised polyarthritis identical to rheumatoid arthritis.

Bone disease whether metabolic, neoplastic or due to Paget's disease may imitate a polyarthritis superficially but careful examination and investigation will always clarify the diagnosis.

Investigations

In the elderly there is no clear cut differentiation between the normal and abnormal: there is a wide grey area of doubt. To use haematological and biochemical investigations in an attempt to establish the diagnosis of rheumatoid arthritis in the elderly, the wide normal limits must be appreciated and results assessed critically.

HAEMATOLOGY

In acute rheumatoid arthritis the haemoglobin level is perhaps as good an indicator of disease activity as is the erythrocyte sedimentation rate. However, it may, in the aged, be an indication of malnutrition or of blood loss from gastro-intestinal lesions such as hiatus hernia, or gastrotoxic drugs. Serum iron levels and iron binding capacity may be helpful in planning treatment but can be influenced by other co-existing disease or drug therapy.

Although diagnostically of little help, except in the rare cases of arthralgia due to the reticuloses, the total and differential white blood and platelet count is important since it may influence the type of drugs to be given. Macrocytic anaemia, sometimes due to folate deficiency, is five times more common in rheumatoid arthritis than in controls (Partridge and Duthie, 1963; Gough *et al.*, 1964). In the elderly this may be confused with pre-existing pernicious anaemia.

BIOCHEMISTRY

Renal function tests are important when the use of potentially nephrotoxic drugs, for example gold or penicillamine, is being considered. They may indicate systemic involvement (but equally may merely reflect the consequences of prostatic obstruction) or chronic pyelonephritis.

Occasionally serum immunoglobulins can be helpful in diagnosis because the degenerative arthropathies and gout are not usually associated with protein abnormalities. Although the tests for the rheumatoid factor are now more specific and a positive result is strong confirmatory evidence of rheumatoid arthritis, it must always be considered with other haematological and clinical evidence lest false positives, which are not uncommon in the elderly, confuse the issue; similarly raised serum uric acid levels may indicate a secondary hyperuricaemia from renal impairment, blood dyscrasias or drugs such as diuretics rather than a primary gout.

If, as often happens, the patient has a positive test for the rheumatoid factor then, unless sodium monourate crystals can be definitely demonstrated from a tophus or synovial fluid, it is safer to assume the arthropathy is rheumatoid. Little harm will result from treating gout as rheumatoid arthritis, because many drugs, for example indomethacin or phenylbutazone, help both but rheumatoid arthritis will never respond to allopurinal or uricosuric drugs, and valuable time may be lost.

RADIOLOGY

Radiology although important is not always as diagnostically helpful as is generally believed, particularly by the patients themselves. Degenerative changes are the rule rather than the exception and may eclipse evidence of an inflammatory arthritis particularly in the weightbearing joint. Peri-articular osteoporosis may be the result of metabolic or senile changes and degenerative cysts may mimic erosions or tophi.

However, serial radiological assessment will provide valuable evidence of the disease's progress and is mandatory where surgery is being considered—in this respect "weightbearing" views are useful in assessing joint stability in the lower limb. The cervical spine, in flexion and extension as well as views of the odontoid peg should not be forgotten when assessing a rheumatoid patient who complains of neck pain or who may need surgery. To ascribe neck pain to "spondylosis" without radiological examination in the rheumatoid patient is a sure way to miss the occasional vertebral subluxation, odontoid erosions and atlanto-axial instability which can materially contribute to pre-existing muscle weakness and loss of mobility.

Treatment

The treatment of rheumatoid arthritis in the elderly is, of necessity, a compromise, determined by the severity of the disease, the patient's age and life expectancy and presence of other coincidental illness.

In the elderly time is at a premium and treatment of a patient with a predictably short life expectancy, whether because of advanced age or incurable disease, must be designed to produce the greatest benefit in the shortest time. Inevitably, this will mean occasionally taking risks which would be unacceptable in an otherwise normal and younger person.

The types of treatment available to the elderly are the same as for the young; medical and physical treatment, rehabilitation in and out of hospital, continuing socio-economic assessment and finally surgery are all part of the total care programme. Most important is the frequent ongoing supervision and an eclectic open-minded approach to drugs particularly the adreno-corticosteroids. The necessity and indications for operation are best discussed at a combined rheumatoid orthopaedic clinic. All surgical intervention is part of the concept of total care and is not to be looked at as an isolated event.

MEDICAL

The primary object of treatment is the relief of pain and the reduction and suppression of the inflammatory reaction to improve function and correct other abnormalities such as anaemia.

Analgesics

These can be conveniently subdivided into those with little or no anti-inflammatory properties, and those which do have such effects.

The most important drugs in the first group are the salicylates. It can be argued that in adequate dosage, these have a significant anti-inflammatory effect. However, prolonged high dosage of salicylates in the elderly is seldom successful because of concomitant deafness, tinnitus and gastrointestinal bleeding (Wood et al., 1962). The concurrent administration of anti-coagulants makes salicylate therapy dangerous. However, aspirin remains the most acceptable of the simple analgesics but should be given preferably as a coated variety or as Aloxiprin to reduce the risk of gastric bleeding to the minimum. It is no longer the sheet anchor of treatment, particularly in the acute rheumatoid arthritis of the elderly, and should not be given to the exclusion of the more potent anti-inflammatory drugs.

Paracetamol and Distalgesic are effective and safe analgesics and, in most patients with rheumatoid arthritis, will give adequate pain relief.

There are many analgesic drugs available nowadays, often offered in combination with other preparations. Despite the claims made in their favour most have little more to offer than the salicylates, and are often more toxic. Generally, preparations containing several ingredients should be avoided in the elderly.

It is advisable to avoid analgesics containing codeine because constipation and old age tend to co-exist, and with active arthritis the physical effort demanded may be such as to jeopardise independence.

The second group of analgesics, with more potent anti-inflammatory properties, contain several well tried and useful drugs, notably phenylbutazone, oxyphenylbutazone, indomethacin and to a lesser extent, ibuprofen. These drugs, particularly indomethacin used as a suppository, are very effective in relieving joint stiffness and decreasing joint swelling. However, there is no convincing evidence that they significantly alter the progress of the disease and they can produce unacceptable side effects.

The coated tablet of phenylbutazone, and liquid preparation of indomethacin do help to lessen the gastro-intestinal effects of these two drugs but they should be avoided in the presence of active gastric or duodenal ulceration. The fluid-retaining properties of phenylbutazone restrict its use in patients with cardiac, hepatic and renal failure; it can also lead to confusion if the ankles and feet are already swollen as a result of local articular inflammation because the condition may appear to have been aggravated. Routine white cell and platelet counts are important because fatal agranulocytosis can occur with this drug.

Indomethacin occasionally produces headaches and unsteadiness (Hart and Boardman, 1963), which appear to be unconnected with the dose level and, unfortunately, recur on further exposure to the drug. In elderly patients with basilar or vertebral artery insufficiency or head and neck pain from cervical spondylosis, these side effects may aggravate their symptoms and the connection of the latter with the drug may not be appreciated.

Both indomethacin and phenylbutazone can be prescribed as suppositories —a very effective method for providing nocturnal relief of pain and avoiding gastro-intestinal disturbance. However, this route of application may be not only unacceptable but impractical, the patient being physically unable to insert the suppository because of joint restriction. Unless the patient is specifically questioned on this aspect embarrassment may result.

The anti-inflammatory drugs

These must form the keystone of the treatment of acute rheumatoid disease in the elderly and should always be considered in the more chronic but active forms. They include gold; the corticosteroids; the immunosuppressive drugs and D. penicillamine.

Gold   Following a multicentre trial in 1960 (Empire Rheumatism Council, 1960, 1961) gold is now an established treatment of definite value, particularly in the early acute cases of rheumatoid arthritis. Carefully monitored it is a safe drug; its most unpleasant toxic effect being pruritis and dermatitis; the most dangerous, renal damage and bone marrow suppression.

There are no hard and fast rules concerning the age limit for gold therapy. In the absence of renal dysfunction, blood dyscrasias or skin lesions, there is no reason why its use should be curtailed although there is probably no place for gold therapy in patients over 70 for whom a more rapidly effective treatment is usually required.

It is usually given weekly by intramuscular injection in doses varying from 10 to 50 milligrammes after an initial test dose to exclude allergy; sodium aurothiomalate is the usual preparation. The clinical response appears unrelated to the blood levels and the duration of treatment still remains undecided. Many physicians, however, do continue to give gold in small maintenance doses for long periods, even over several years.

Among the disadvantages of gold therapy are the need for regular urine analysis and leucocyte and platelet counts, frequent injections, and the latent period, often six weeks or more, before clinical improvement occurs. For an elderly person incapacitated by acute arthritis, and who is, perhaps, living alone, this latent period may be unacceptable. It is, therefore, vital to provide adequate supportive treatment possibly in hospital during this period.

Although psoriasis often remains unaffected by gold therapy, other dermatoses may be aggravated. The elderly are very prone to skin disorders and careful examination, particularly of the flexures and interdigital areas is important. The pruritis and rash caused by gold may often persist for months and can be very distressing.

Systemic corticosteroids   The indications for using this group of drugs are still wide and subject to varying interpretations and prejudices. They have an ill reputation which is probably overemphasised and dates from the days when large doses of the less sophisticated preparations were used indiscriminately. There can be no argument concerning their potential toxicity and their prescription needs to be carefully monitored. However, one fact is definite; this group of drugs will, in adequate dosage, produce a more rapid suppression of the inflammatory process in rheumatoid arthritis than any other anti-inflammatory drugs (Medical Research Council and Nuffield Foundation 1959, 1960).

For this reason alone, corticosteroids are extremely important in the treatment of rheumatoid arthritis in the elderly, when time for more conventional treatment is limited. Many elderly people, particularly those living alone, exist on a knife edge, their independence and mobility threatened by any change in social or medical status. An acute inflammatory arthropathy represents a very real danger.

Corticosteroid therapy should be considered as the first line of attack in any patient over 70, and possibly in the over 65 age group where adverse social and economic factors are present. In some patients the drug may be given as an interim measure until other methods of treatment help to control the disease. In most patients a permanent maintenance dose will be needed. This should be as low as possible and related to the patient's functional ability and clinical state rather than pain, which can usually be controlled by analgesics.

Obviously, in the presence of gastro-intestinal disease, either a coated and soluble preparation should be used or it should be given by injection. If the maintenance dose is low, then fluid retention and Cushingoid features will be very slight. Unfortunately, in the elderly bruising and tearing of the skin, particularly over the lower legs and forearm, can be a problem sometimes producing ulceration. The patient should be advised to wear protective clothing, such as shin guards made from thin foam plastic worn under stockings or tights to act as a buffer and to prevent the skin being broken by any slight injury.

Osteoporosis with vertebral collapse often occur in the elderly but these are not such common complications of corticosteroid therapy as was at first thought. Stress fractures can also occur, especially in the leg bones (Devas, 1975).

Unless corticosteroids are used on a short term basis to provide immediate cover until other measures take effect, they will be required permanently. The consequences of sudden cessation of these drugs and the problems associated with intercurrent illnesses, especially gastro-intestinal upsets, should be fully explained to the patient and immediate relatives and the patient should be provided with an appropriate "steroid" card.

A.C.T.H. and the synthetic anterior pituitary hormones are not very suitable for the elderly because of their high incidence of side effects and the need for frequent injections.

Local corticosteroids Intra-articular injections of corticosteroids are extremely valuable (Hollander *et al.*, 1961) and, in the patient with few affected joints, may obviate the need to give more potent oral preparations. Even in patients with many affected joints, rapid relief can be obtained by this procedure. Frequently, tendon sheath lesions in the palms cause loss of hand function. These resolve in most patients after local corticosteroid infiltration, forestalling an unnecessary surgical intervention.

Destructive changes in weightbearing joints have been reported in a few cases of rheumatoid arthritis after repeated intra-articular corticosteroid injections (Chandler and Wright, 1958; Sweetnam *et al.*, 1960). There is still some doubt whether this is a true complication of the injections or due to the natural disease process. However, it is wise for patients to avoid excessive mobility for a few days after intra-articular injection of corticosteroid into weightbearing joints and injections should be restricted to once every three or four weeks. The suppressive effect upon the adrenals must be remembered, since there is good evidence that this may persist for up to seven days even with the short-acting corticosteroids (Shuster and Williams, 1961). The dangers of infection following intra-articular injections have been exaggerated and are very uncommon when a sterile technique is observed. It is a safe, effective treatment which can be provided equally as well in the patient's home as in the consulting room or hospital.

D. penicillamine   This drug, a chelating agent, has been used for a number of years in the treatment of rheumatoid arthritis but only over the past five years has its value been appreciated. Several trials suggest it will become an important noncorticosteroid drug in treating early acute cases although the mode of action is not understood (Andrews *et al.*, 1973). As with all effective antirheumatic drugs, it has its share of side effects, principally dyspepsia, loss of taste, bone marrow depression, renal and hepatic dysfunction.

Provided patients are adequately screened beforehand there appears to be no reason why it should not be used in the elderly. It must be given in gradually increasing doses and possibly an upper limit of 900 milligrammes of penicillamine hydrochloride or its equivalent base should not be exceeded. The patients must be assessed often for proteinuria, haematuria and white cell and platelet depression. Less regular blood urea estimations and liver function tests are important. As with gold there is usually a latent period of some weeks before clinical improvement occurs, the patient therefore requiring other supportive treatment in the meanwhile.

Immunosuppressive agents   The two most frequently used in the treatment of rheumatoid arthritis are azothiaprine and cyclophosphamide. They are both effective and there is evidence that erosive changes may be reversed. At present they are mainly given either in an attempt to reduce corticosteroid dosage or for the severe complications of rheumatoid arthritis such as arteritis. However, their use is being expanded to cover the acute early case. They are not drugs to be prescribed where hospital cover is unavailable because leucocyte suppression is the rule rather than the exception; renal and liver damage can also occur. Carcinogenesis and infertility are long term complications but can be safely ignored in the elderly.

Gold, the corticosteroids, D. penicillamine and the immunosuppressive drugs are all potentially dangerous but effective drugs in the treatment of rheumatoid arthritis. In the elderly, with fragile renal, hepatic and gastro-intestinal systems, these drugs must not be prescribed without full clinical, social and economic appraisal. The risks must be assessed against possible improvement, over what will in many cases be for only a few years. Risks unacceptable in the young, may be ignored for such benefits.

Other drugs

Active rheumatoid arthritis is commonly accompanied by anaemia, often hypochromic and normocytic in type. However in the elderly, inadequate nutrition, occult bleeding from hiatus hernia, B_{12} or folate deficiency may complicate the haematological picture. Whatever the aetiology, appropriate drugs should be given to rectify the anaemia. In rheumatoid arthritis, oral iron appears to be less effective than intramuscular or intravenous preparations (Richmond *et al.*, 1958). In severe cases with active disease whole blood transfusion can be very useful.

The most effective way of raising the haemoglobin level in patients with rheumatoid disease is by controlling the disease.

The elderly are often malnourished and suffer from avitaminoses because of economic pressures. Therefore it is reasonable to prescribe vitamin supplements, particularly Vitamin C. Insomnia because of nocturnal pain is debilitating and can be relieved by careful use of sedation.

PHYSICAL

Physical therapy should not be divided into physiotherapy and occupational therapy but considered as part of total care and rehabilitation, the object being to relieve pain, improve function and mobility by physical measures. These measures must be directed to the general good of the patient rather than improvement of a particular joint.

The elderly patient presents special problems, general assessment and an agreed planned programme being essential before treatment is started.

Needs and limitations

The essential requirement of the elderly patient is independence of toilet, feeding, dressing and mobility around the home. Obviously, mobility outside the home is important but because the perimeters of many elderly people are voluntarily restricted, this is of less importance than the needs listed above.

Assessment of daily living activities is, therefore, the first task of the therapist, not only in the rehabilitation department but also in the patient's home. The help of the spouse or a relative should be enlisted so that an accurate picture of the patient's "day" can be obtained.

From this information a programme combining pure physiotherapy, such as heat, shortwave diathermy or ultrasound designed to relieve pain, can be combined with exercises related to normal creative work performed in the occupational therapy department. Motivation in the elderly is often poor and, if the patient is given stereotyped exercises after a course of heat and left in a cubicle unattended, the inevitable result is boredom and sleep. Group therapy does encourage a degree of competition and is usually acceptable and often enjoyed by an old person who may lead a lonely existence.

Active exercise may be restricted or contra-indicated by the presence of cardiovascular, respiratory or neurological deficiencies. The therapist will not be thanked for precipitating congestive failure by over-enthusiastic treatment. It is essential for the therapist to be aware of the patient's overall clinical state and where possible to be included in case conferences.

Although many rehabilitation departments treat the young and elderly together, this may be to the detriment of the latter, whose pace is slower, and who may become confused by noise. Therefore the elderly may respond better to individual treatments.

The journey to and from a rehabilitation department, particularly in rural areas, can be exhausting and time consuming. It is better for the elderly to attend on a whole day basis and provision of a day centre or hospital in close proximity to the therapy department is very useful. Day centres should be mandatory where new units are being designed. Hydrotherapy is extremely well tolerated and enjoyed by young and old. In the latter it enables joint movements to be executed with the least effort.

Provided they are made and fitted carefully, splints can provide considerable comfort and can prevent deformity if worn conscientiously. Although tolerance does not increase with age, the patient may be more co-operative if the rationale is explained fully. If the patient's skin is thin due to the arthritis or corticosteroids the splints should be made from a softer plastic material such as Plastazote rather than plaster. Velcro straps are easier for the patient to handle than leather with buckles. Above all the therapist must be sure that the patient can put on the splints without help or has help at home to do so.

Knee cylinders are never very satisfactory, whatever the material, particularly in the very unstable joint. Generally, if a knee is so damaged that a cylinder is necessary then a replacement arthroplasty should be considered.

Walking aids are frequently incorrectly prescribed, or sometimes completely forgotten. The elderly patient is often reluctant to use a stick because of appearances and the implication of infirmity. However, tactful explanation will often produce a change of mind and acceptance of a walking aid.

Elbow or gutter crutches, if necessary custom built, are preferable to sticks because they provide greater stability by spreading the load over the whole upper limb rather than concentrating pressure in the hands and wrists. In the home most disabled, elderly patients prefer walking frames which can be adapted to carry household items and do not need to be propped up against furniture and walls.

Wheelchairs may not be necessary in the home but they are needed if the patient is to escape into the outdoor world from the immediate environment. Careful prescription is imperative and the medical condition of the relative likely to propel the chair ascertained because he or she will, in most cases, also be elderly and equally subject to cardiac, respiratory or locomotor disease.

Electrically driven chairs, particularly the type with independent wheel drive and micro-switch control, for use in the home are sometimes more practical than self-propelling models. If necessary both types can be prescribed for indoor and outdoor use.

It is unusual for the elderly arthritic patient to be eligible for a motorised invalid car. However, there is no reason why a vehicle should not be modified, if one is owned.

SOCIAL
It is advisable for all elderly patients with rheumatoid arthritis to be assessed

by a medical social worker. Most will need support whether it is in the nature of "Meals on Wheels", home help or recuperative holidays. Ongoing social care is as important as continuous medical care and must involve close co-operation with the relatives, whose burden is frequently underestimated, as well as with their medical attendants.

The importance of orthopaedic surgery cannot be over stressed in the elderly. It is surprising how apparently "poor risk" patients survive and benefit from major orthopaedic procedures such as replacement arthroplasties which involve relatively short periods of immobility and hospitalisation.

Surgery

The object of orthopaedic surgery in elderly patients with rheumatoid disease is to relieve pain and improve function. By so doing independence may be retained or restored and the quality of life enriched. To obtain the best results careful planning before and after operation is essential.

The patient with well controlled disease or in remission can be treated in much the same way as an ordinary geriatric orthopaedic patient. However, where active rheumatoid disease exists then not only must the nature of the proposed operation be carefully considered but also the timing of the operation, the need for physical therapy beforehand, the stabilising of drug dosage (particularly if corticosteroids are being taken), the duration and type of rehabilitation afterwards and, finally, a firm proposal of the date of discharge home.

If such planning is to be successful there must be a multidisciplinary approach. Usually the patient will have been referred by either a rheumatologist or the family physician. Nevertheless an up-to-date assessment of the general condition is as important as the orthopaedic lesions, but no patient, however disabled or ill, should be denied the opportunity to be considered for surgery. There is no merit in improving a patient's locomotion if the presence of poor respiratory function or cardiac ischaemia will neutralise the benefits of, for example, a replacement arthroplasty. However, most surgeons with experience of surgery in the elderly rheumatoid patient will agree that risks, unacceptable in the younger patient, are worth taking and are usually gladly accepted by the patient so that continued independence may be enjoyed.

It is helpful to have a full medical social worker's report and the assessment by the therapists is of particular value.

Because so many aspects of the patient's condition must be considered and because time is valuable, combined clinics and care conferences can be very instructive and helpful, enabling decisions to be made rapidly.

Many elderly patients with rheumatoid disease are in what may be termed "injury time" and cannot have their admission delayed, as would be the case if their names were put on a routine surgical waiting list. The latter will ensure that many will never live to benefit from operation. If a rheumatoid patient needs an orthopaedic operation, it is needed at once. The condition may deteriorate so rapidly that, after six months the proffered operation may have no benefit.

At Hastings this problem is overcome by having a special list of patients who may either be admitted to the orthopaedic ward directly or from the rheumatological ward after a period of preparation, to which they return a day or two after operation.

The operation, as in all geriatric surgery, must be considered as one incident in the total care of the rheumatoid patient, although an important incident. Therefore, before operation the patient is brought up as an out-patient for specific therapy not only to the part concerned but in general both to improve the patient as a whole and to allow a full assessment of the capabilities. This is necessary in order to know what the patient needs to be independent at home.

Patients with rheumatoid disease are particularly prone to infection not only at operation but also metastatic infection; therefore it is necessary to delay operation until any small septic focus has been treated and healed.

PREPARATION
The operation must be done under the strictest aseptic measures. Before operation the skin is carefully prepared in the usual manner and antibiotic cover given; in our experience one of the cephalosporins gives the best results.

THE OPERATION
If the patient is going to have any form of operation during which blood loss will occur or afterwards if a pneumatic tourniquet has been used, blood must be available to replace the blood loss and to maintain a normal haemoglobin level during convalescence.

The operation must be done with proper speed to avoid unduly long exposure of the tissues; this helps to avoid wound infection. After operation suction drainage is used to prevent haematoma formation.

The day after operation the patient is got out of bed to enable return to the rheumatology ward the next day where monitoring of the general condition is done by the rheumatologist. This means that the operation done must have been chosen so that the patient can continue at once with rehabilitation in just the same way as does the ordinary geriatric patient.

CHOICE OF OPERATION
The elderly rheumatoid patient may present a greater challenge than the geriatric patient with ordinary osteoarthritis because of the many parts affected by the rheumatoid condition. Very often careful planning is

necessary to ensure that the proper sequence of operations is used, so that rehabilitation can proceed. Thus a patient needing both a hip and a knee replacement should have the knee done first because it is easier to use crutches or a walking frame with a bad hip than with a bad, and often unstable, knee.

The upper limbs, after a hip or knee replacement, will be used for a walking aid probably more than before operation for the first few days and the assessment and treatment before operation will have been directed to this. It may, on occasion, be valuable to treat a troublesome elbow before doing joint replacements in the leg.

Occasionally the severity of an arthritis makes operation urgent, such as the sudden and complete collapse of the head of the femur in an osteoporotic patient with rheumatoid disease. However, this must not prevent the full assessment of the patient before operation.

The fracture near the hip in a patient with rheumatoid arthritis does demand special consideration. It has been said that elderly patients who have a fractured neck of femur should have a replacement, while the young patient should have the fracture fixed internally. In the patient with rheumatoid arthritis this indication for replacement occurs at a much younger real age, but the physiological age is of course, older.

In general the surgical procedures done for the elderly rheumatoid arthritic patient are the same as for any other old person, but often needing greater urgency and there need be no fear in replacing joints at a somewhat younger age. The rationale for this is that the mileage to be done on any one joint will be limited by the disability as a whole.

As is so often the case in dealing with geriatric problems, a full and close association between the rheumatological and orthopaedic departments so that each may understand the problems of the other will ensure that the patients get the best out of any surgical procedure with the least complication and the shortest time in hospital.

References

Andrews, F. M., Golding, D. N., Freeman, A. H., Golding, J. R., Day, A. T., Hill, A. G. S., Camp, A. V., Lewis-Fanning, E. and Lyle, W. H. (1973). Controlled Trial of D(-) Penicillamine in Severe Rheumatoid Arthritis. *Lancet* **1,** 275.

Bartholomew, L. E. (1965). Isolation and Characterisation of Mycoplasms (PPLO) from Patients with Rheumatoid Arthritis, Systemic Lupus Erythematosus and Reiter's Syndrome. *Arthritis and Rheumatism* **8,** 376.

Bermann, R. R. and Jillson, O. F. (1961). Hyperuricemia and Psoriasis. *Journal of Investigative Dermatology* (1961) **36,** 105.

Blumberg, B. S. (1960). Genetics and Rheumatoid Arthritis. *Arthritis and Rheumatism* **3,** 178-185.

Bremner, J. M. and Lawrence, J. S. (1966). Population Studies of Serum Uric Acid. *Proceedings of the Royal Society of Medicine* **59,** 325.

Chandler, G. N. and Wright, V. (1958). Deleterious Effect of Intra-Articular Hydrocortisone. *Lancet* **2**, 661-663.

De Blecourt, J. J., Polman, A. and De Blecourt-Meindersma, T. (1961). Hereditary factors in Rheumatoid Arthritis and Ankylosing Spondylitis. *Annals of Rheumatic Diseases* **20**, 215.

Devas, M. B. (1975). "Stress Fractures". Churchill, Livingstone, Edinburgh.

Dixon, A. St. J., Beardwell, C., Kay, A., Wanjka, J. and Wong, Y. T. (1966). Polymyalgia Rheumatica and Temporal Arteritis. *Annals of Rheumatic Diseases* **25**, 203.

Duthie, J. J. R., Stewart, S. M., Alexander, W. R. M. and Dayhoff, R. E. (1967). Isolation of Diphtheroid Organisms from Rheumatoid Synovial Membrane and Fluid. *Lancet* **1**, 142-143.

Empire Rheumatism Council. (1950). Report on an Enquiry into the Ecological Factors associated with Rheumatoid Arthritis. *Annals of Rheumatic Diseases* **9**, Supplement.

Empire Rheumatism Council. (1960). Gold therapy in Rheumatoid Arthritis: Report on a Multicentre Control Trial. *Annals of Rheumatic Diseases* **19**, 95.

Empire Rheumatism Council. (1961). Gold therapy in Rheumatoid arthritis: Report on a Multicentre Control Trial. *Annals of Rheumatic Diseases* **20**, 315.

Gough, K. R., McCarthy, C., Read, A. E., Hollin, D. L. and Waters, A. H. (1964). Folic-Acid Deficiency in Rheumatoid Arthritis. *British Medical Journal* **1**, 212-217.

Hart, F. D. and Boardman, P. L. (1963). Indomethacin: A new Non-Steroid Anti-inflammatory Agent. *British Medical Journal* **2**, 965-970.

Hollander, J. L., Jesser, R. A. and McCarthy, D. J. (1961). Synovianalysis: An Aid to Arthritis Diagnosis. *Bulletin of Rheumatic Diseases* **12**, 4, 263-264.

Lawrence, J. S. and Ball, J. (1958). Genetic studies in Rheumatoid Arthritis. *Annals of Rheumatic Diseases* **17**, 160.

Lewis, J. G. (1961). Gout and the Haemoglobin Level in Patients with Cardiac and Respiratory Disease. *British Medical Journal* **1**, 24-26.

Medical Research Council and Nuffield Foundation. (1959). Comparison of Prednisolone with Aspirin on other related Analgesics in Rheumatoid Arthritis. *Annals of Rheumatic Diseases* **18**, 173.

Medical Research Council and Nuffield Foundation. (1960). Comparison of Prednisolone with Aspirin on other related Analgesics in Rheumatoid Arthritis. *Annals of Rheumatic Diseases* **19**, 331.

Partridge, R. E. H. and Duthie, J. J. R. (1963). Incidence of Macrocytic Anaemia in Rheumatoid Arthritis. *British Medical Journal* **1**, 89.

Richmond, J., Roy, L. M. M., Gardner, D. L., Alexander, W. R. M. and Duthie, J. J. R. (1958). Nature of Anaemia in Rheumatoid Arthritis. *Annals of Rheumatic Diseases* **17**, 406.

Short, C. L., Bauer, W. and Reynolds, W. E. (1957). "Rheumatoid Arthritis". Harvard University Press, Cambridge, Massachusetts.

Shuster, S. and Williams, I. A. (1961). Adrenal Suppression due to Intra-articular Corticosteroid Therapy. *Lancet* **2**, 171-172.

Steinberg, P. G., Becker, S. W., Fitzpatrick, J. B. and Kierland, R. R. (1951). A Genetic and Statistical Study of Psoriasis. *American Journal of Human Genetics* **3**, 267-281.

Sweetnam, D. R., Mason, R. M. and Murray, R. O. (1960). Steroid Arthropathy of the Hip. *British Medical Journal* **1**, 1392-1394.

Wood, P. H. N., Harvey-Smith, E. A. and Dixon, A. St. J. (1962). Salicylates and Gastro-Intestinal Bleeding: acetylsalicylic acid and aspirin derivatives. *British Medical Journal* **1,** 669.

Ziff, K., Schmid, F. R., Lewis, A. J. and Tanner, M. (1958). Familial Occurrence of the Rheumatoid Factor. *Arthritis and Rheumatism* **1,** 392.

7

Arthritis in the Elderly

C. G. ATTENBOROUGH

The Hip and Knee

Osteoarthritis and rheumatoid arthritis of the hip and knee are most disabling orthopaedic conditions, particularly in an elderly person. The pain and stiffness caused by these conditions inevitably cause a steady slowing up, loss of function and consequently an increased difficulty in the activities of daily living. Added to this, the knee especially may become insecure either giving way and allowing the patient to fall, or by laxity of the ligaments and subsequent deformity, making the patient fearful of trusting it. Many elderly people live alone, often moving to upstairs accommodation. As pain and stiffness increase, such patients are less and less able to go out of doors to do their shopping, less able to use any form of public transport and more dependent on relatives or neighbours. Gradually they become housebound. Even if they do not live alone, it becomes increasingly difficult to move around their home. Housework becomes too difficult, morale sinks and eventually the patients become chair or even bed bound. They have suffered a total loss of independence.

Arthritic conditions of the hips and knees can often be bilateral and indeed frequently both hips and both knees can be involved either simultaneously or in various combinations. Bilateral disease of the hip or knee can be a very serious disability but equally severe may be the involvement of one hip and one knee on the same side or one hip and the opposite knee.

It is fortunate that orthopaedic advances in therapeutic methods, including the total replacement of joints, have so improved the outlook for such grossly disabled patients that it is now often possible to alleviate the pain and disability, to return confidence in movement and function and thus enable them to regain their independent existence.

Early Treatment

The conservative management of both rheumatoid arthritis and osteoarthritis in its early stages is well known, including the use of sticks and pain relieving drugs. The judicious use of proper physiotherapy can also be helpful, but under no circumstances should these measures be prolonged once the patient is losing function or suffering pain which is more than just a nuisance.

DRUGS

For the patient with rheumatoid arthritis, a full assessment should be made by a rheumatologist (see Chapter 6) who will prescribe the necessary drugs. For the patient with osteoarthritis Indomethacin 25 milligrams three times a day seems particularly helpful in early osteoarthritis but its dangers, especially of gastric bleeding, should be borne in mind.

OTHER MEASURES

In both diseases some simple physical measures may help. Many patients can be helped by persuading them to use one or even two sticks, by losing weight, by adjusting the height of their shoe to correct shortening and, at the same time, using a rubber heel to act as a buffer when walking on hard surfaces. In the physiotherapy department short wave diathermy is often helpful in relieving some of the pain and active muscle building exercises are of great importance and proprioceptive neuromuscular facilitation methods appear to be the most valuable particularly in the stage of treatment immediately before operation. These consist essentially of resisted exercises with very little movement, bringing into use both the muscles concerned and their antagonists.

In the physiotherapy and occupational therapy departments the patients can also be greatly helped by an assessment of their activities of daily living and supplying them with any aids which may be necessary to help them retain their independence.

Conservative methods often may keep the patients going for many years with relatively minor disability but it must be emphasised that the geriatric patient on the whole is no less a candidate for operative treatment for osteoarthritis and rheumatoid arthritis than is any other age group. Once the point of continuing disability has been reached, with the inability to achieve a satisfactory quality of life, the indication for operation is present and, in a geriatric patient, is often more urgent than it might be in a younger age group.

Surgical Treatment

INDICATIONS

Pain and loss of function are the main indications for operation on patients with osteoarthritis or rheumatoid arthritis. Severe, spontaneous pain is an obvious indication for operation, but, if the pain is severe only on weight bearing and is relieved by rest, then the patient must be assessed on the loss of function for, as Devas (1974) has so strongly emphasised, loss of function in the elderly often means loss of independence. Age is no bar to the replacement of a joint provided the patient is carefully assessed beforehand and the necessary medical measures taken to treat the concomitant diseases that more often than not co-exist in the elderly patient. Nonagenarians are by no means to be excluded; many have had a successful joint replacement, sometimes bilaterally, and returned to an independent life in which the quality of existence has once again become acceptable.

Operation should never be postponed in the elderly. If there is any doubt as to whether it is now indicated or not, then the operation should be done. This is because the old person will rarely make an improvement in general health. The inactivity produced by an added disability, such as a painful hip of knee, causes a general loss of muscle tone and may prevent the patient leaving home which will lead to further ill health from malnutrition.

THE HIP

In the past the results of operations have been unpredictable. The long period of rehabilitation needed after vitallium mould arthroplasty of the hip precluded its use in many elderly patients. Partial replacement of the hip using a Thompson or a Moore prosthesis allows a quicker rehabilitation but the degree of relief of pain is uncertain and a recurrence of symptoms often follows. Such operations should be abandoned in the elderly. The place of intertrochanteric osteotomy in the treatment of osteoarthritis is still to be decided. It may still be the treatment of choice in younger patients. In some centres osteotomy is still recommended for the old person provided that the radiographic appearance of the hip does not show that the condition is far advanced. Results, however, are unpredictable and it is our practice never to use intertrochanteric osteotomy in the treatment of osteoarthritis or in rheumatoid arthritis in the elderly. When it has been decided that an operation is needed, then it must be a total hip replacement which is the best and most satisfactory operation for the elderly patient.

THE KNEE

Excision of the patella may often be of great value if it is the patello-femoral compartment that is mainly involved; this is rarely found to be the case in patients with rheumatoid arthritis. Osteotomy of the upper end of the tibia or of the tibia and lower end of the femur has in its unpredictable results much the same disadvantage as the intertrochanteric osteotomy in the hip. In our view it should never be undertaken in rheumatoid arthritis and rarely, if at all, in osteoarthritis in the elderly. It used to be the practice at Hastings to do a high tibial osteotomy, with early walking thereafter and without restriction of knee movement (Devas, 1969), but this has now been superseded in the elderly patient by total knee replacement. This operation has been used for many years but it is only recently that a sufficiently reliable and satisfactory method has been produced so that it can be used as a routine procedure in geriatric orthopaedics.

Thus, total knee replacement, having lagged behind total hip replacement, has few long-term results, but even so they are very encouraging provided the correct technique is used.

ASSESSMENT BEFORE OPERATION

Once it has been decided that a joint replacement is needed to alleviate the pain and disability of an arthritic knee or hip, the patient's general health must be carefully assessed. A full blood count must be done, the haemoglobin content estimated and respiratory, cardiovascular and renal function must be assessed. This is best done in consultation with an anaesthetist and a geriatrician as described in Chapters 2 and 3. The patient with rheumatoid arthritis must be assessed in consultation with the rheumatologist. This is mandatory for all major surgical procedures on patients with rheumatoid lesions needing joint replacement. Before operation it is best for the patient to be admitted to a combined rheumatological orthopaedic unit. Whether or not physiotherapy has been given previously, the patient must be under the supervision of a physiotherapist for at least one to two weeks before operation. During this time the ability to walk, to rise from a chair and to manage stairs is carefully noted; resisted exercises are started for all muscle groups.

This treatment before operation has been found to increase the speed of rehabilitation after operation, particularly for the knee, whether it be for osteoarthritis or rheumatoid arthritis. The exercises are continued on admission to hospital so that the patient will know exactly what is needed of her after operation.

It is our practice to give routine antibiotic cover starting before operation and continuing thereafter, using cephaloridine 500 milligrams intramuscularly with the premedication and repeating this six hourly until the patient can take 500 milligrams of cephalexin orally four times a day. This is continued for at least one week after operation. We believe that this may contribute to a reduction of late sepsis, which in our hands has been very low even before the use of the ultra clean air Charnley Howarth unit.

TECHNIQUE OF OPERATION

The hip

At Hastings both the Charnley and the McKee Arden procedures are used, the choice being individual to the surgeon. It would be superfluous to describe here the operative details of total hip replacement. Surgeons have their own preference for surgical approach but we believe that the antero-lateral approach used for the McKee Arden operation and the lateral approach for the low friction arthroplasty as described by Charnley, in each case using the technique described by the originator, give the best results. Dislocation after operation has been rare and this we attribute especially to the avoidance of the posterior exposure. The posterior skin incision may also make infection more likely, being much closer to the anal region and to the pressure areas when the patient is lying.

The knee

Design   The first generation of implants for total knee replacement were the hinged joints. The Shiers and the Waldius are probably the best known examples. These allow flexion and extension but are totally restrained from all other movements. They impart great mechanical stability to the knee but the restraint necessary to give this stability makes them vulnerable to torsional strain and loosening of the components in the bone is a very real problem.

In order to overcome this the surface or condylar prostheses were produced as the second generation. These consist of liners for the femoral and tibial condyles which are unconnected and nearly unrestrained and therefore less prone to disruption of the cement-bone bond. However, because of their lack of inbuilt stability they are unsuitable for patients with more than a minor degree of instability or deformity.

The problem, therefore, has been to design an implant which has stability but which does not loosen in bone with torsional strains. Two such joints have been designed at Hastings. The "link" arthroplasty has overcome the problem by setting the femoral component between the femoral condyles thus preventing rotation, and, because no joint surface is excised, preserving the collateral ligaments intact. So far, loosening has not been a problem. The main disadvantage was the fact that it was a metal-to-metal weightbearing implant; as such it is unsuitable for the younger geriatric patients and must be confined to the very old. It imparts an excellent degree of stability and allows a good range of movement (Fig. 1).

The second knee produced at Hastings has been the Stabilised Gliding Prosthesis (Fig. 2). It has been designed as a compromise between the restrained hinged joint and the unconnected surface prosthesis, being a two-piece implant allowing the normal gliding movements of flexion and extension with a stabilising rod between the femoral and tibial components, which allows some lateral mobility and rotation but acts in place of the cruciate ligaments and in place of or in addition to the collateral ligaments. This implant has a cobalt-chrome femoral component and a high density polyethylene tibial component and is, therefore, suitable also for a younger age group.

Biomechanical considerations   The load on the knee has been investigated by several engineers, notably Morrison (1967), Harrington (1973) and Paul

(1974). It has been shown that in normal level walking a load of the order of three to four times body weight is carried mostly through the medial condyles in the weightbearing phase. This load rises to nearly five times body weight during ramp and stair ascent and descent. The lateral condyles carry a load during the swing phase mainly due to muscle contraction. In an arthritic

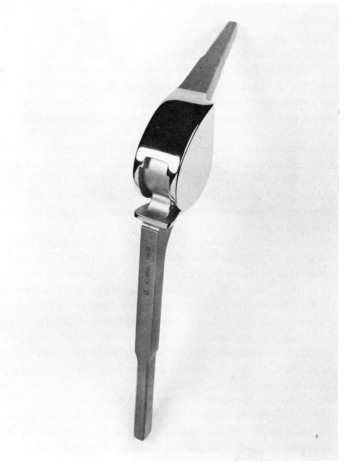

FIG. 1 Devas "Link" Knee Prosthesis.

patient with an undeformed knee these loads may be much reduced because of the lower level of activity but when the knee is deformed the load may increase considerably, particularly on the ligaments. In normal walking the anterior cruciate ligament is active chiefly during the early part of the stance phase soon after heel strike, whereas the posterior cruciate transmits forces mainly during the latter part of the stance phase and, of course, when descending stairs and ramps. The collateral ligaments take less load except when the knee is deformed.

The patello-femoral joint has not been considered in the design of many total knee prostheses. It must be remembered that the patello-femoral joint carries a load of about half body weight in level walking but this rises to nearly three times body weight in ramp descent.

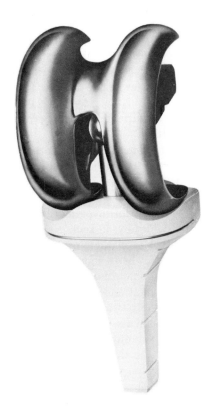

FIG. 2 The Attenborough Knee Prosthesis showing the stabilising rod.

Torsional strains are considerable in walking but the rotational forces in other activities must also be considered. With a straight knee, turning to the right or left with the foot fixed to the ground produces a high torque on both the femoral and tibial components of a restrained hinge joint. If the knee is bent then most of the rotational strain will fall on the tibial component but when a lateral force is applied, the femur will be the more affected. Rising from a chair or getting out of a car are examples of movements which involve both lateral and rotational strains.

The hinged total knee prostheses are extremely stable but it is probably this very stability which predisposes to loosening when torsional and lateral strains are applied. The surface or condylar prostheses, of which there are now many examples, are unconnected and therefore nearly unrestrained and should, therefore, be less likely to disruption of the cement-bone interface by these torsional and lateral strains. However, they are certainly not immune from loosening and this may be in part due to retention of the cruciate ligaments. The likely cause of this is discussed later. These implants rely for their stability on intact ligaments and are, therefore, unsuitable for patients with a major degree of instability or deformity, and it may well be that their indication is primarily in early but painful disease.

There are, therefore, certain criteria which should be met in the design of an implant for total knee replacement. It is desirable that weight should be taken through the condyles, as in the normal knee and not through the intercondylar region. A load in the intercondylar region may make stress fractures more likely, particularly in the osteoporotic bone of a patient with severe rheumatoid arthritis.

Flexion and extension movements should approximate to the normal knee. Ideally all other movements should be unrestrained so that the danger of loosening of the prosthesis is kept to a minimum with lateral and torsional strains. No built in restraint at all would be necessary in an operation on a normal knee but in a severely arthritic patient there is often much instability and sometimes a severe deformity; in such cases an unrestrained prosthesis will give rise to an unstable and therefore an unsatisfactory knee. Total restraint as in the hinged prostheses should be avoided and a compromise is necessary. The design should allow normal rotation and lateral laxity so that some of the strain of torsional and lateral strains are removed from the cement-bone interface. Some restraint is also necessary to control antero-posterior and lateral movements, particularly in full extension so that stability is preserved when standing and walking.

The length and shape of the stem should be carefully considered. A long stem has the disadvantage that a later salvage procedure with removal of prosthesis and cement, for instance in a case of sepsis, means that the femur and tibia may have to be guttered for a considerable distance to remove all the cement and infected material. There is little doubt also that long stems with long columns of cement may damage the blood supply of the cortex of the femur and tibia over a considerable distance and this too may make loosening more likely. A short or absent stem on a prosthesis may be satisfactory in a totally unconnected surface prosthesis but in an implant with some built-in restraint then a stem is required. There seems little point in taking the stem beyond the dense cancellous bone as the cement has less bonding value to cortical bone. There should probably be a stem of about 75 millimetres tapered to drive the cement into the trabeculae of the cancellous bone and with sufficient cross section to give a large surface area of contact between cement and bone.

There is a widely held belief that the cruciate ligaments should be retained. This may not be correct. In a severely diseased knee, destruction of cartilage and bone may bring the tibial spines into contact with the intercondylar region of the femur, producing a flexion deformity which cannot be overcome without removing the tibial spines and thus the cruciate ligaments. This is the reason why many surface prostheses cannot be used in cases with more than a few degrees of flexion deformity. If a surface prosthesis is used in a less damaged knee there will be an abnormal differential tightening of one or other retained cruciate ligament unless the exact dimensions of the lower end of the femur are reproduced in every case. This is impossible with most surface prostheses and the abnormal tightening of the cruciates may produce an antero-posterior shearing force leading to component loosening.

The design of the prosthesis should call for the removal of a minimal length of bone so that a secondary procedure can still be performed in case of failure. Probably less than 2 centimetres of bone length should be removed.

Most designs for total knee replacement have failed to take into account the patello-femoral joint. There is an increasing number of patients with patello-femoral pain after a so called total knee replacement. The patello-femoral joint should be replaced.

In the light of our present knowledge metal-to-plastic joints should be used in weightbearing implants. These give a bearing with less friction making loosening less likely. Recent work has suggested that the wear debris in metal-to-metal joints gives rise to sensitivity to one or other of the constituent metals and it is believed that this may predispose to loosening of the component. The wear debris in these joints has also been found to be carcinogenic in rats and there are some cases reported of malignancy arising in human hip joints. Whether or not these are coincidental or connected in any way remains to be seen.

The stabilised gliding prosthesis   The stabilised gliding prosthesis is one of the third generation of knee implants (Fig. 2). It has a femoral component made in chrome-cobalt alloy. This consists of shells for the two femoral condyles attached to a tapered intramedullary stem 75 millimetres in length (Fig. 3). At the base of the stem is a hollow into which is fitted a ball on the end of a rounded stem (Fig. 2). The ball is free to rotate and its stem runs in a gap between the posterior parts of the femoral condyles. This gap is just greater than the stem's diameter in front and therefore restricts lateral movement in extension. The gap widens at the back, allowing the stabilising stem to move from side to side. The weightbearing surface of the prosthesis has a radius of 40 millimetres and there is a smaller radius of 25 millimetres posteriorly and anteriorly. These latter two curves are long enough at the back to allow flexion of the knee through more than 90 degrees and in the front to enable the patella to articulate with the femoral prosthesis in all positions of the joint.

The tibial component is made in high density polyethylene and has a tapered hollowed intramedullary stem 70 millimetres in length, into which fits the stem of the femoral component. The tibial plateau is shaped with a radius which is the same as the larger 40 millimetre radius of the femoral condyles (Fig. 3). Thus in extension the two components fit exactly and,

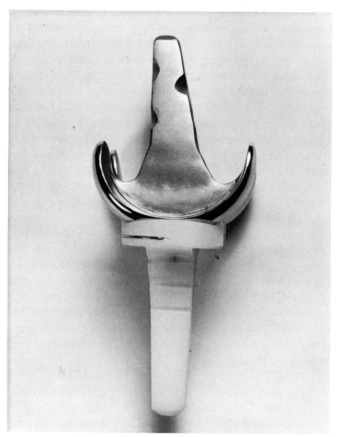

FIG. 3 Attenborough Stabilised Gliding Knee Prosthesis.

under load, rotation is controlled. As flexion increases the smaller curve of the posterior parts of the femoral condyles comes into apposition with the tibial plateau (Fig. 2) and some backward and forward movement of each femoral condyle is possible allowing rotation. The tibial surfaces are so shaped that as rotation occurs the joint opens tightening the soft tissues and preventing over-rotation. Some of the strain is thus taken from the cement-bone interface. In flexion too, the stabilising rod is in the widening gap between the condyles of the femur and able to move sideways allowing some lateral mobility which increases with flexion and decreases to nothing in full extension mimicking the normal knee. Once again with lateral movement the joint opens allowing the soft tissues to take some of the strain. The tibial stem is hollowed to a greater depth than the length of the stabilising rod to allow for any wear which may take place between the femoral and tibial condylar components.

The movement in this prosthesis is polycentric because of the variable curve of the femoral condyles. The length of the stabilising rod projecting below the condyles must therefore vary according to the position of the joint (Fig. 4). Thus in extension there is a longer projection than in flexion. This makes the rod move up and down within the tibial component. This movement has been harnessed to improve the lubrication of the joint. There is a hole drilled from just below the weightbearing surface of each side of the tibial plateau to the bottom of the central hole containing the rod (Fig. 5). The rod has one flattened surface. Synovial fluid can run into the bottom of the central hole when the knee is flexed and in extension the rod acts as a piston driving the fluid up again and out through the two small lateral holes close to the main weightbearing surfaces and around the shaft of the stabilising rod itself.

Each component has a relatively short tapered stem with a large cross section. The design of the implant is such that the bone length which has to be removed is limited to between 1 and 1.5 centimetres.

Preparation   Before operation the patient is treated with resisted exercises with minimal movement to strengthen the quadriceps and hamstrings, and is also taught the hamstring and quadriceps exercises for after the operation.

Operation   The patient is placed in the supine position and a pneumatic tourniquet is used. Exsanguination is by elevation. An Esmarch bandage tends to damage the skin of a patient with severe rheumatoid disease.

A straight lateral parapatellar incision is used and the skin is reflected medially deep to the deep fascia to allow the joint to be opened on the medial side. The criticism of this type of valvular incision is that it may predispose to necrosis of the skin on the medial side. This has not been our experience. The incision has several advantages. If there is any delay in skin healing and this, of course, is not infrequent in rheumatoid arthritis, the joint itself is not exposed and this limits the direct entry of any superficial sepsis to the joint. The lateral skin incision also avoids damage to the infra-patellar branch of the saphenous nerve which is so frequently divided by an incision on the medial side leaving an area of numbness over the front of the knee joint. When correcting valgus deformities it is often necessary to divide the lateral retinaculae in order to centralise the patella. This is very simple through the lateral skin approach.

The knee joint is opened through an almost midline incision in the quadriceps down as far as the superior pole of the patella and then skirting

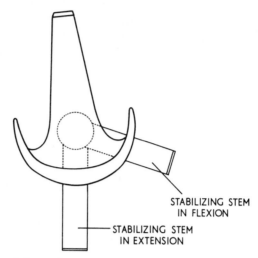

FIG. 4 Diagram of femoral component showing linking stem in extension and in flexion.

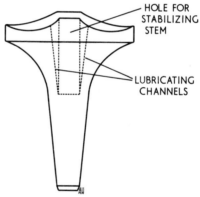

FIG. 5 Diagram of tibial component showing hole for stabilizing stem and lubricating channels.

the medial side of the patella and ligamentum patellae, leaving enough soft tissue attached to the patella for suturing at the end of the operation. The knee joint is now flexed fully, dislocating the patella laterally. This should be done slowly and under direct vision and, in a case of rheumatoid arthritis with a previously very stiff knee, adhesions may have to be divided and sometimes also the cruciate ligaments in order to avoid bone damage, particularly to the tibial spines when obtaining full flexion.

About 1 centimetre of bone length is removed from the femoral condyles, making the cut at right angles to the axis of the lower femur in the lateral view and parallel to the femoral condylar articular surface in the antero-posterior view (Fig. 6). If, however, one or other of the femoral condyles is badly collapsed, then the direction of the cut in the antero-posterior view must be such that it leaves the cut bone at about 7 degrees of valgus in relation to the axis of the shaft of the femur. When the patient has a severe valgus or varus deformity, it should be remembered that in most instances the deformity is because of collapse of one or other of the tibial condyles and allowance for it is made in inserting the tibial prosthesis.

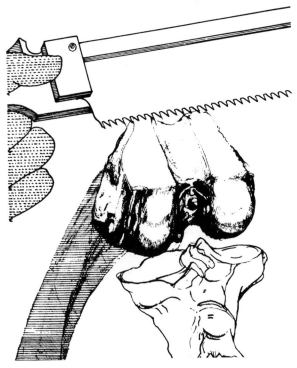

FIG. 6 Removal of 1 centimetre of bone length from lower end of femur.

Using the femoral template, a rectangle of bone is removed to open the medullary cavity of the femur and this is then deepened just sufficiently to allow the insertion of a femoral trial instrument (Figs 7 and 8). The posterior surfaces of the femoral condyles are removed flush with the back of this instrument. In large-boned individuals the anterior surface may have to be trimmed in line with the front of the instrument, particularly when osteophytes are present, but as little bone as possible is removed from the front in order to preserve the integrity of the femoral condyles. The anterior and posterior corners are removed with a saw so that the lower end of the femur now roughly fits the rounded inner surface of the femoral prosthesis.

The anterior cortex of the femur between the condyles is removed to a depth of 0.5 centimetres and the posterior cortex to a depth of 3 centimetres from the cut surface of the femur to allow the femoral prosthesis to recess fully and the stabilising rod to move into a fully flexed position without coming into contact with the posterior cortex of the femur.

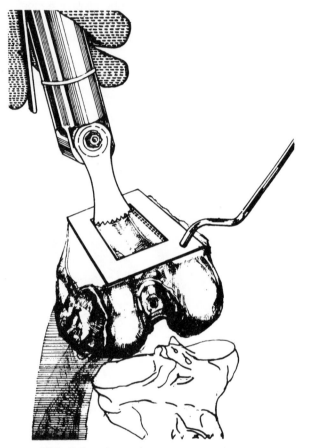

FIG. 7 Opening medullary cavity of femur.

The knee is fully flexed to expose the tibial plateau. If necessary the femoral trial instrument can be left in position to protect the cut bone and the tibia held forwards using a bone lever behind the upper end of the tibia and levering against the femoral trial instrument. The raised tibial spines are removed but it is not necessary to remove the whole of the upper surface of the tibia and indeed as much as possible of the hard subchondral bone should be preserved. The line of section of the upper end of the tibia is very important. In the lateral view it should not necessarily be parallel to the tibial plateau as this often has a posterior inclination and if the section is parallel a flexion deformity will result. The bone should be divided at right angles to the axis of the shaft of the tibia in the lateral view. Seen from the front, the line of section should also be at right angles to the axis of the tibia and this will correct any valgus or varus deformity.

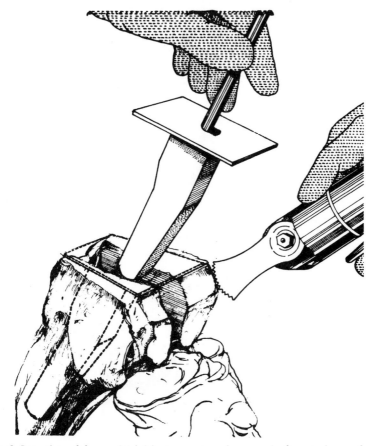

FIG. 8 Insertion of femoral trial instrument and removal of posterior surfaces of femoral condyles.

Using a tibial template, a rectangle of bone is removed from the cut surface of the tibia and at the upper end of the tibia and the lower end of the femur it has been found that the use of an oscillating saw limits the likelihood of splitting of the condyles (Fig. 9). Cancellous bone is removed until the tibial trial instrument can be inserted with the stem exactly in the long axis of the tibial shaft (Fig. 10). In both the femur and the tibia the removal of cancellous bone should extend only just deeper than the trial instrument in order to avoid cement being forced a long way down the medullary cavities.

A trial fit is now undertaken using a femoral prosthesis and the tibial trial instrument with its handle removed. Residual valgus, varus or flexion deformity can be corrected, if necessary, by removing a little more bone from the lower end of the femur. It is important to test flexion to at least 100 degrees to make sure that there is sufficient clearance to avoid the

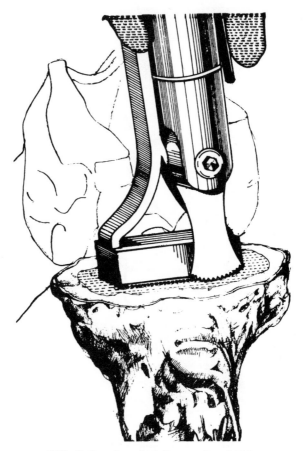

FIG. 9 Opening medullary cavity of tibia.

stabilising rod coming into contact with the posterior surface of the femur.

With the knee fully flexed the tibial prosthesis is cemented in, using an introducer. Cement is allowed to fill any gap between the upper tibial surface and the underside of the prosthesis. Cement is then placed in the medullary cavity of the femur and the trial femoral instrument is inserted to approximately half its length removing any excess cement which bulges posteriorly. Before inserting the femoral prosthesis some cement is used to line the inner surface of the condyles of the prosthesis and a pack of absorbable gelatine

sponge is placed behind and around the stabilising rod to prevent cement
entering the back of the prosthesis during insertion. The prosthesis is then
inserted into the femur, at the same time allowing the stabilising rod to enter
the hole in the tibial prosthesis. The knee usually needs to be flexed to just
beyond a right angle and straightened to a right angle as soon as the

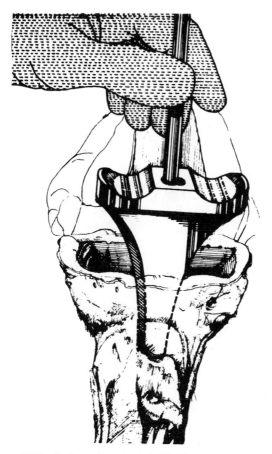

FIG. 10 Insertion of trial tibial instrument.

prostheses are linked. The femoral prosthesis is held securely in position
while the knee is gently flexed to the fullest possible extent and then brought
back to a right angle (Fig. 11). This pushes excess cement backwards and
this can be helped by the use of a Macdonald dissector pushing the bulging
gelatine sponge backwards and clearing any remaining sponge from within
the prosthesis. The knee is now fully extended and this keeps a very firm
pressure on the femoral prosthesis while the cement hardens. Once hard the
knee should be tested again in flexion and it may be necessary to trim some

cement from the outer side of the femoral prosthesis. At this stage also the lateral retinaculae may have to be divided to make sure that the patella can be centralised easily. The incision is now closed using suction drainage and, as the patient will be encouraged to start early flexion of the knee, it is important to suture the deep fascial and subcutaneous layers securely,

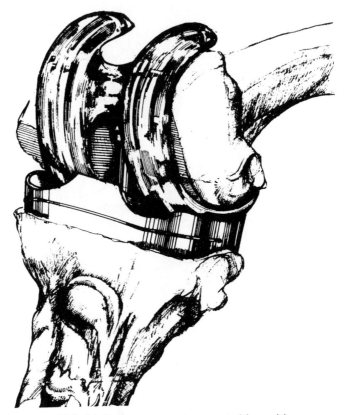

FIG. 11 Both components cemented in position.

particularly in rheumatoid arthritis where there is a danger of delay in skin healing. A wool and crepe pressure bandage is applied. No plaster is necessary. The ease and rapidity of mobilisation of patients after inserting this prosthesis has been a feature of its use.

Care After Operation

With a total joint replacement of either hip or knee most geriatric patients need two or three units of blood during or after operation. After hip replacement the intravenous infusion is continued so that half a litre of dextran can be given daily over the next three days. This is in an endeavour to reduce the incidence of deep vein thrombosis and pulmonary embolus. Suction drains and, for the knee, pressure dressings are removed at 48 hours. All patients, after both hip or knee replacement operations, are out of bed and helped to walk on the day after operation. Thereafter they are out of bed for a longer time each day. The psychological benefit to the elderly patient in being allowed to sit out of bed soon after operation in our opinion contributes materially to a rapid return of function and to independence. Despite early mobilisation, pressure sores may occur unless precautions are taken. The care of the skin must be scrupulously maintained in the same way as described in Chapter 9 on hip fractures.

Joint movements are started on the day after operation and it is essential that all patients after hip and knee replacements should continue the resisted muscle exercises that were taught before the operation. After knee replacement flexion of the knee is allowed as far as is comfortable but in patients with severe rheumatoid arthritis and abnormal skin, flexion should not be encouraged beyond 45 degrees until the skin is known to be soundly healed.

Most of the patients are fit to be transferred to their homes or a convalescent home at one week from the date of operation and their sutures are removed either by the district nurse or at the convalescent home at 12 to 14 days, or longer in severe rheumatoid disease. Some of the very frail and elderly patients, particularly those who develop some other medical condition, are transferred to the geriatric orthopaedic unit a few days after operation to continue their rehabilitation. Some patients, in whom a condition such as a previous hemiplegia complicates the operation, are transferred as a matter of principle. Patients with rheumatoid arthritis are returned to the rheumatological orthopaedic unit 48 hours after operation. Once the patient leaves hospital little or no physiotherapy is needed after a total hip replacement but after a total knee replacement some patients may need supervised physiotherapy until their quadriceps and hamstrings are redeveloped and until they have regained the fullest flexion possible. Within a few weeks most patients will have discarded walking aids in favour of one stick when walking out in the street and this also is often discarded a short while later.

Complications

INFECTION

Prevention of infection is best achieved by a meticulous surgical technique which involves both ward and theatre nursing staff. The use of antibiotic cover and the ultra clean air Charnley Howarth unit, have resulted in a negligible amount of immediate infection after operation. In the rare cases of late infection we endeavour to control this by antibiotics over a long period but, occasionally, after total hip replacement the prosthesis and cement have been removed, leaving a pseudarthrosis. The design of both the prostheses used at Hastings for total knee replacement is such that, after removal of the implant and cement, an arthrodesis can be satisfactorily achieved with no shortening of note.

DEEP VEIN THROMBOSIS

Deep vein thrombosis is a relatively common problem after total hip replacement and we have normally treated this by using anticoagulant therapy though the value of this is still in dispute. Pulmonary embolus is still the main cause of early death after a total hip replacement but this too, fortunately, has been rare in our series. In total knee replacement deep vein thrombosis has been conspicuous by its absence and there has been no case of death from pulmonary embolus.

Conclusion

There is little doubt that total hip and total knee replacement are two of the most significant advances for many years in the treatment of disabled geriatric patients. These techniques have enabled many hundreds of patients to avoid a wheelchair or bed bound existence and thus retain their independence. A word of warning is, however, indicated. Some patients after operation on a joint which has restricted their activities to a marked degree have regained the ability to be very much more mobile. There are instances where this increased mobility has precipitated in rheumatoid arthritis the rapid disintegration of another joint and, in both rheumatoid arthritis and osteoarthritis, there are instances of severe post-operative intermittent claudication because of the increased ability to exercise and, in the same way, severe angina or even death from coronary thrombosis can occur.

A further finding is that some patients, who have been unable to walk because of one painful hip or knee, develop a stress fracture, usually of the opposite femoral neck, from the great increase in activity that the replaced joint now allows.

Other Joint Replacements

In osteoarthritis it is rarely necessary in a geriatric patient to replace joints other than the hip and the knee. In rheumatoid arthritis, however, arthroplasty may be required in several other joints, notably the shoulder, elbow, wrist and ankle. The indications for these are the same as for rheumatoid arthritis at a younger age group. The final answer to joint replacement in these joints has not yet been found but biomechanical and clinical research has produced several shoulder and ankle prostheses which are now under trial, but we must await long-term follow-up results. In the case of the wrist joint, an arthrodesis may often be the treatment of choice but in an elderly person when both wrist joints are involved, an arthroplasty will often be desirable. Several wrist joints are under trial including a stabilised gliding wrist joint produced at Hastings.

The elbow joint has many of the problems of the knee joint in that stability is required but total restraint from all movement except flexion and extension is undesirable. Many of the elbow joint prostheses so far produced have been of the hinged type and the humeral components have shown a marked tendency to loosen in the bone. This is almost certainly due to rotational strain in a prosthesis with no rotational laxity. As in the knee, there are now some implants which are of the condylar and, therefore, totally unconnected types but these are still in their trial phase. At Hastings the problem has been approached in a similar way to the knee, but the link elbow in which the humeral component fits between the condyles has, after several years, shown problems of loosening. However, the stabilised gliding elbow replacement appears to have the same merits as does the similar knee replacement.

Acknowledgements

Figures 4 and 5 Reproduced by permission of Mechanical Engineering Publications Ltd.

Figures 2, 3, 6, 7, 8, 9, 10 and 11 reproduced by permission of Annals of Royal College of Surgeons of England.

References

Devas, M. B. (1974). Geriatric Orthopaedics. *British Medical Journal* 1, 190-192.
Devas, M. B. (1969). High Tibial Osteotomy for Arthritis of the Knee—A Method specially suitable for the Elderly. *Journal of Bone and Joint Surgery* 51B No. 1.
Harrington, I. J. (1973). Knee Joint Force in Normal and Pathological Gait. M.Sc. Thesis, University of Strathclyde, Glasgow.
Morrison, B. B. (1967). The Forces Transmitted by the Human Knee Joint During Activity. Ph.D. Thesis, University of Strathclyde.
Paul, J. J. (1974). Force Actions Transmitted in the Knee of Normal Subjects and by Prosthetic Joint Replacements. *Institution of Mechanical Engineers* C271/74.

8

Fractures in the Elderly. Introduction

MICHAEL DEVAS

In the following chapters the principles of fracture treatment in the elderly will be described with particular emphasis on management and operative techniques that have been found useful or that differ from the usual methods used in other age groups.

Table 1 shows a comparison of the total elderly population in the Hastings area and the United Kingdom as a whole.

In order to achieve a proper orthopaedic service to this elderly population very intensive methods of treatment and management are necessary for success; this applies to the in-patient and out-patient alike.

In treating old people restoration of function is, as usual, the most important aim; but to them it means a return to independence. The latter is jeopardised by a long stay in hospital and bed rest in itself is dangerous and should be as short as possible. Walking is the most necessary function in maintaining independence and must be achieved at the earliest possible moment.

Table I

COMPARISON OF AGES IN THE HASTINGS DISTRICT AND IN THE
UNITED KINGDOM*

		POPULATION (in thousands)					
		Aged 65 and over		Aged 65 to 74		Aged 75 and over	
	Total	No.	%	No.	%	No.	%
Hastings Health District	145	39.7	27.4	23.4	16.2	16.3	11.2
United Kingdom	55,610	7,203	13	4,214	7.6	2,989	5.4

*Based on Census 1971, County Report, East Sussex; DHSS 1974, Health and Personal Social Services Statistics for England (1972) figures) and Census of Population Reports.

In the treatment of fractures in the elderly certain techniques which are suitable at younger ages have been abandoned because of failure to restore independence quickly; thus many weeks in traction for a fracture of a femoral shaft has given way to methods of internal fixation that allow the patient to walk immediately even though such a course would be unacceptable in youth.

In the treatment of fractures near the hip the results of simple pinning were poor, especially when compared to the far easier management of the patient after a cemented replacement of the femoral head. This emphasises that it is the patient who has to be treated and not the part for although a united fracture of the neck of the femur will, when satisfactory, give a better hip than one with a femoral head replacement, the patient as a whole does better with the latter.

Similar intensive care and treatment should be given to the elderly with fractures who do not need admission to hospital; the fracture clinic must be geared to careful surveillance of the patient from the time of the injury to discharge; this in fact cuts down the time the patient continues to attend. The old lady with the Colles's fracture will have daily treatment to prevent stiffness and osteoporosis in the affected limb and to preserve the muscle tone until the plaster is removed, when the movements of the wrist and other parts will be sufficiently good to allow the patient to continue exercises at home.

Fractures near the hip are the most important problems to solve in any district where there are many elderly people. Without a proper concept of the management not only will patients with such fractures, but all other geriatric patients with severe injuries, languish in hospital unnecessarily long to their own detriment, to the frustration of the medical staff and to cause a poor ward turnover. Thus, it is still heard that old people with fractured femora are blocking beds. This is a criticism of management and not an excuse. Age is not the fault of the patient, nor does the patient wish to remain in a hospital bed but is instead only too anxious to be up and independent. Contrary to the opinion of some who believe that the old are only too happy to lie in a warm ward with instant attention and with three meals a day, such patients are almost invariably anxious to return to the most simple accommodation that is "home", where they may live a life of independence which will compensate for all the other inconveniences that a meagre purse may necessitate.

The technique of treating fractures near the hip is dealt with in a separate chapter because of its great importance, not only to the individual patient, but to the orthopaedic unit concerned. Proper management of a patient with such a fracture will lead to early discharge from hospital and early return to independence; it will prevent the many complications consequent upon undue decubitus, it will result in proper and thus much increased usage of beds in an acute orthopaedic ward. Financially, it is more economical to support an old person at home than in an old people's home or, worse, in a long stay geriatric bed. With the increasing age of the population it is imperative that everything should be done that can be done to maintain the independent existence of all old people and that a heavy initial expense be considered as a sound investment financially. Far more important is the quality of life of the patients who will invariably wish to remain independent at home, to live out their lives in their particular way.

General Principles

The bones of an old person not only break easily but also unite readily. Whatever the fracture, the patient must be reassured as soon as possible that all will be well, that the broken bone will heal and that function will be restored. Osteoporotic bone unites in exactly the same way as does ordinary bone and no less quickly. Osteoporosis should not be considered as a pathological process but as a physiological withdrawal of bone strength.

The importance of osteoporosis in a geriatric patient lies in the fact that simple decubitus increases the calcium loss and therefore the bone strength; at the same time when any part, such as a leg, is immobilised the effect is compounded. Therefore the aim of fracture treatment in the elderly must be to obviate the fracture and to allow the patient to walk forthwith. The choice of the treatment of a fracture in an old person must be taken seriously and it is a responsibility that should never be delegated; included in the treatment is a proper after care service and the latter is, in a sense, far more important than the technical achievement of fixing the fracture at operation.

Any elderly patient who comes to hospital with a fracture, but with no clear history of the fall or injury that caused it, must be investigated carefully on several counts: first some old people sustain a drop attack or a similar collapse which, for no apparent reason to them, lands them on the floor in their own home with no history of slipping, tripping or stumbling. These injuries hold a very bad prognosis, not so much for the part broken but for the integrity of the patient as a whole. Often such a fracture is a symptom of the impending dissolution of the patient. The system is beginning to disintegrate and the patient is suffering, literally, from old age. The occurrence of a pathological fracture must never be forgotten; and, especially in the femoral neck, some stress fractures can become complete so that the fracture has occurred before the patient falls.

Other fractures occur in patients who are about their daily business, walking in the street, hanging up their laundry or otherwise enjoying an active existence. In these patients one expects a far better prognosis than in the group described above; usually the fracture has been caused by considerable violence. When the fracture is near the hip it will be found, more often than not, that the patient in falling or slipping has in fact hit the ground in such a way that the hip was directly involved and the fracture was not caused by a torsional force passing upwards from a rotation strain on the lower leg. The activity of this group of patients is the key to treatment, that is, to keep all geriatric patients with fractures as active as possible.

Should an active person of advanced years attend with some injury for which there was no real violence and which from experience in that type of patient should not have caused the damage, then great care must be taken in making sure that the diagnosis of a simple fracture is correct and that it is not a pathological fracture. These will be obvious in the case of Paget's disease with which there may well be a history of bone pain. It may not be so obvious if there is a localised weakness because of a malignant condition. Myelomatosis must always be remembered because it is comparatively common in old age. A generalised myelomatosis may not show clearly on the radiograph and the small amount of bone absorption caused by the condition and evenly distributed may well be missed if the radiograph taken at the time of admission is not of the highest quality. If proper enquiry as to the cause of the fracture is not made valuable weeks or months may be lost before the correct treatment is given.

In an old person who is active it is quite possible to get a stress fracture. This should be treated in the same way as in a younger age group but with greater attention to certain parts such as the hip in which, if the one develops a stress fracture which needs treatment then it is likely that the other may have a similar stress fracture hidden and symptomless.

Often the old, but active, person who develops a stress fracture, for example in the tibia, and having been told that there is a broken bone, will believe that there must have been some injury. Such patients may then inculpate a slight trip or jar some time previously as the cause of the broken bone. This is because the patient cannot accept that there is a break in a bone without a cause; careful enquiry may well reveal that the ache that was present before the visit to hospital for the radiograph was also present before the trivial injury.

It is, therefore, essential that all elderly people suffering from a fracture have a history taken carefully so that no important point may be lost. This should be normal practice at all ages but, regrettably, too often the diagnosis is made radiologically and not clinically. Once an obvious fracture has been seen it is accepted for what it is and as the result of an injury.

Having established the diagnosis and the cause of the fracture it is important to assess the patient's background and the circumstances in which she lives. It is necessary to find out exactly what is needed for the patient to continue to be able to live outside hospital, either at home or in sheltered care while the fracture is uniting. It is quite impossible for an octogenarian to live alone in a flat or apartment with many stairs and with no help if one ankle is in a below knee plaster on which the patient cannot bear weight. It can be very difficult even if only one wrist has a Colles's fracture and is in plaster. Even more disabling is the impacted fracture of the neck of humerus which, even though needing only a sling and active rehabilitation, may so disable the patient that existence without help cannot be managed. It is all part of the total care of the geriatric orthopaedic patient to ensure that the proper attention is given to the circumstances of the patient; in the same way that younger patients are always asked about work, so should geriatric patients always be asked about the circumstances in which they live.

There must be a careful assessment of the prognosis because many old people are fortunate to have a relative who may come and live with them for a period of time. If, as in the case of a Colles's fracture, it can be guaranteed that the plaster will be removed in four to five weeks and that thereafter the function will be satisfactory and the patient restored to her condition before the accident, then firm plans can be made and often help is forthcoming. Again, relatives of the patient with the more incapacitating fracture near the hip, they will accept responsibility when they know that the patient will be in hospital for only two or three weeks and thereafter will need some help at home for a short while. It is to be emphasised to relatives or friends of such patients that the condition is not a disastrous and final interruption of independence but one that is only temporary; it is best considered as one of the many inconveniences that beset the elderly that will be put right in a very short time.

After the less severe fracture, the elderly patient is usually fit to go home later the same day after the fracture has been set under a general anaesthetic and put into a plaster cast. A misplaced feeling of pity or other emotional reaction must not influence the decision to send the patient home or to cause the patient to be admitted to hospital. Nothing could be worse. Age alone is no indication for admission to hospital and under no circumstances should admission be merely for rest. The old person has an eternity of rest to follow and to be admitted to hospital to do nothing is the worst possible treatment that could be devised. The whole concept of return to function after a fracture, not only in the elderly but at any age, is activity to maintain muscle tone. To put a geriatric patient into a ward to be rested in bed or in a chair for the whole of the day means that the muscle tone is lost in the quickest possible way and, with it, osteoporosis will increase and the patient will leave hospital in a worse state than she entered it.

The proper indication for admission to hospital is the complete loss of independence of the patient. The aim of admission will be the restoration of function and with it the restoration of independence as quickly as possible. Once the necessity for admission has been decided, it is then important to consider which method of treatment will enable the patient to get home quickest. Often the answer is internal fixation, but this is not always so. Thus the elderly lady with bilateral Colles's fractures may need to be in hospital because she is unable to manage her personal toilet. Again, an above knee walking plaster is satisfactory for a young, active man who can use crutches with little trouble but such treatment is completely disabling to the octogenarian; then the decision must be made as to whether that patient is fit for conservative treatment or should have internal fixation to allow immediate and unencumbered walking.

A good example is the patient with a fractured neck of humerus. This is a common fracture in the elderly and usually is impacted. Often a simple collar and cuff sling outside the clothes is sufficient treatment and most patients are able to manage even if they live at home. However, in some the pain of the fracture is so great that all activity is curtailed and admission to hospital inevitable. This is an indication for immediate internal fixation which is neither difficult nor risky and takes only a few minutes to do. The next day the patient will be up and about, function in great measure will have been returned and with it independence so that return home is possible.

To admit such a patient and not to operate would be wrong because the pain is again sufficient to prevent all activity except to sit out of bed, which is usually the most comfortable position, so that to lie in bed is more painful than to sit; unfortunately the patient is not allowed to sit out of bed all night and so it is possible for the general condition to deteriorate because of admission to hospital.

It is to be accepted that there is a definite indication for internal fixation of fractures in the elderly even when the fracture would unite satisfactorily with conservative treatment. There must never be any hesitation in eliminating external splintage that immobilises the patient or prevents the independent activities of daily living and, instead, substituting internal fixation, which will allow early walking, the fracture having been eliminated and leaving only the wound to heal. Even so, great care must be taken not to subject a patient to some form of open reduction which does not allow immediate activity because then the patient has to recover from both the fracture and the operation.

The treatment of a fracture is only a small part of the care of the geriatric patient and once the injury has occurred there will always be the necessity for rehabilitating the whole patient. Many old people when seen at hospital for some injury are found, for example, to have bronchopneumonia, hypertension, vertebro-basilar insufficiency or multiple small cerebrovascular accidents, any one of which may cause a momentary giddiness or loss of full awareness so that the patient falls. Every out-patient must have a proper investigation before being allowed home.

After a geriatric out-patient has had a fracture treated and has returned home it is necessary to have a proper system of continued care to prevent the patient not doing the necessary exercises for the limb concerned as well as continuing to do all the activities of daily living. One of the worst things that can happen to an elderly out-patient with an arm in plaster is to have a relative who takes it upon herself to nurse the patient, to the detriment of the part concerned which remains stiff after the plaster has been removed. It is as important as at any other age that the limb should be kept fully functional in the parts not actually immobilised. This, and other problems, will be prevented by adjusting the normal follow-up routine of a fracture clinic specifically for the elderly.

At Hastings, for the first few days after a reduction of a fracture the elderly out-patient will have special attention in the physiotherapy department to control swelling and start movements. As soon as the swelling is better, usually in two or three days, the patient is transferred to the occupational therapy workshop where she will be given a task adjusted for that type of injury so that the whole limb is used. In this way, function throughout is maintained, tone is kept up even in the muscles immobilised by the plaster and osteoporosis is less severe than otherwise. At the time when the cast is removed it is found that most elderly people have both a sufficiently good muscle tone and range of movement in the previously immobilised joint so that they may be discharged from the fracture clinic. A sling, in the same way as over zealous care by a relative, must be discarded as soon as possible because it makes the patient think it proper not to use the arm and the disability is increased in the minds of others so that as much as possible is done for the patient, to her great detriment.

The geriatric patient with a fracture must get a safe and stable result with satisfactory function to allow continuing independent existence but there is no need to insist on the patient regaining a full range of movement that she may not need for the activities of daily living and which, if insisted upon, would cause unnecessarily long remedial treatment; this can be detrimental to the patient and costly to the department. Long continued attendance for therapy will, over the months, exhaust a geriatric patient and, which is perhaps more important, produce a feeling of disability and failure. Further, a slight deformity after a fracture is of little consequence to the old person who is far more concerned with a quick return to function rather than a perfect appearance. Treatment by repeated manipulation or even operation will usually mean that it will take much longer to restore function than if the deformity was accepted (Pool, 1973). The quick return to function far outweighs the theoretical risk of arthritis developing in the far distant future to which no geriatric patient can look forward.

Fixation of Fractures in the Elderly

Old bone unites as well as young bone but osteoporotic bone, even though it joins up in the normal way does not give the same purchase to mechanical fixation as does the young, mature adult bone. It is therefore important to remember certain applications of the principles of bone fixation which are of great value in dealing with fractures in the elderly.

One of the most important techniques to be used is that of always tapping the hole drilled in bone to take the screw. Self tapping screws are excellent for general use but once a bone has become osteoporotic to any degree and therefore the amount of bone less than in the normal, there is to each turn of the screw less bone to grip the thread and so it is easy either to over screw or cause loosening by having drilled too large a hole by movement of the drill in the operator's hands: this will occur even when the correct drill size has been chosen for the screw concerned. It is our practice at Hastings always to drill bone in an old person with the correct size of drill for the screw followed by tapping the drill hole and then inserting the screw carefully to ensure that the thread of the screw meets the thread tapped in the bone and that it does not become cross threaded or, in any other way, damage the bed prepared for it.

Another application which must be remembered is that the old person is rarely as strong as the mature adult and consequently forms of fixation may, at times, be used which would not necessarily be trusted in a young and healthy adult in early life. For example, sometimes a fracture in the upper femoral shaft will be satisfactorily held in place by a pin and a seven (or twelve) hole plate; provided there is good purchase by at least four of the screws below the fracture it is perfectly safe to get the ordinary geriatric patient walking forthwith. The muscle tone will not be sufficiently strong to cause bending or loosening of this form of internal fixation whereas in a young adult further immobilisation would be needed; it is well known that in youth an intramedullary nail may be bent purely by muscle power. This will not happen in the geriatric patient. So fixation must be secure but it need not necessarily have the same rigidity as for youth; nevertheless great care must be taken to assess each patient and to make sure that the fixation used will be satisfactory.

Osteoporotic bone may require plating in one form or another and when this occurs and when the screws appear not to grip well despite all the precautions mentioned above, then it is satisfactory to use a high density polythene plate (Gallannaugh, 1974) on the opposite side of the bone to the rigid metal plate. The polythene plate can be used for one or more screws as necessary.

High density polythene plates

High density polythene has been used very successfully as one half of a joint replacement and because it has been well tried there has been no compunction in using it in other forms. Normally high density polythene for prosthetic inserts must be sterilised by methods other than heat but when high density polythene is to be used in a manner in which it will only need to preserve its strength for a few weeks, it has been found satisfactory to autoclave it before use.

The high density polythene plate can be cut to shape with bone forceps. The plates are about 15 millimetres wide and 3 millimetres thick. When they are applied no holes need to be made for the screws. This is done by holding the plate against the bone in the proper place and, with a drill of one or two sizes smaller than that used for the bone, a hole is drilled through the polythene. The first non-selftapping screw is then inserted, it will engage in the polythene plate and will pull it tightly against the bone with such compression that no further tightening is possible. Once the first screw is in position the next hole is drilled in the polythene plate in the same way.

If too big a hole is drilled into the polythene the screw can pull out. There is no necessity to tap the hole in the high density polythene plate.

We have found this procedure of very great value, particularly in fractures of the long bones of the leg where absolute fixation is essential in the osteoporotic bones of the frail patient. Severe osteoporosis makes it imperative to allow the patient out of bed the following day and, with this technique, it is achieved with greater safety than heretofore.

Sometimes in smaller fractures which are disabling to a patient, such as the broken medial malleolus, simple screwing would be sufficient if a proper purchase could be got in the small malleolar fragment; often it is too soft in texture to allow this, but if a high density polythene washer is cut to shape and placed between the screw and the surface of the malleolus, the screw will not split the bone but obtain good compression and fixation.

INDICATIONS FOR INTERNAL FIXATION

The ordinary indications for operative reduction and fixation of any fracture apply to the elderly in the same way but over and above there are many special indications.

Perhaps the first and most important is that the fractured neck of femur in the geriatric patient should have an immediate prosthetic replacement and not internal fixation. This is based on the experience over many years in treating an ever increasing number of elderly patients with such fractures. All elderly patients with fractures are best treated by the immediate restoration of function and, where bone continuity cannot be safely restored at once, as in the femoral neck, then replacement is the best treatment of the patient. It is our practice to attempt to treat all younger patients conservatively, including traction and bed rest for as long as is necessary; such treatment in a geriatric patient is contra-indicated because of the morbidity it entails. Age in itself is an indication for surgical intervention and fixation.

There is no point in operating on a patient if thereafter the patient has to recover from the fracture as well as the operation. Under no circumstances should any procedure be done for a fracture which does not allow the patient to be up and walking the next day, with the fracture to be disregarded because it has been securely dealt with.

PLASTER CASTS

Plaster casts must always be considered carefully before use. In the upper limb it is more acceptable than in the lower limb. A plaster cylinder extending from the ankle to groin can be tolerated by an old person and walking is safe with the aid of a walking frame. If a plaster cast includes the whole foot with a rocker, heel, or at best a thin soled plaster overboot, then the patient may experience considerable difficulty in walking, to the extent that living at home alone is impossible.

Therefore in certain injuries it is preferable not to enclose necessarily the joint above, or below, the fracture. If a geriatric patient attends with a small but painful fracture in the upper tibia a simple plaster cylinder from above the ankle to the groin may well allow the patient to remain independent and able to look after herself at home. A full length walking plaster would severely handicap such a patient.

The treatment of the fracture must be considered only in the context of the treatment of the whole patient and, if the treatment for the part is bad for the whole, then it must be discarded in favour of another, which is satisfactory to both.

Reduction of Fractures

In reducing fractures under a general anaesthetic which is our routine and which is preferable to a local anaesthetic in this age group, the end result in terms of long term arthritic changes to a joint damaged by the fracture do not have to be considered in the same way as in youth. It is remarkable how a damaged, and slightly deformed, joint will become painless and useful by early movement and remain so thereafter.

It is important in this context to consider the "mileage" of the patient because this will then emphasise that the wear and tear on the joint is going to be very slight compared to that in healthy adult life. A patient retired from work at 65 will walk approximately the same mileage on the hip or knee between the years of 65 and 70 as she would have been done between the years of 30 and 31. A 70 year old will probably do, in her next ten years, less mileage than she would have done in six months as a teenager. Consequently the wear and tear on a damaged joint is going to be slight, particularly if the patient is physiologically old and frail.

Shortening after a fracture in the old person need neither be criticised in the same way as it might be in the younger adult, nor have excessive attempts at its prevention. Osteoporotic bone can be so soft that the fractured ends may compress so that despite their end-to-end reduction there is some shortening. Spiral fractures treated by internal fixation may remain with some shortening. Provided this is not more than 2 or 3 centimetres it is easily accommodated by a differential raise on an ordinary shoe. Most women, and it is in women particularly that fractures occur, object at any age to a clumsy shoe. To compensate for shortening of 2 or 3 centimetres the heel on the good leg should be lowered by one third of the amount of shortening and the heel on the short leg raised by the same amount. This leaves one third of the shortening not compensated; this is usually of little consequence. The patient is satisfied that the shoes are not ugly and morale, always so important, is encouraged.

Preparation for Operation

The care of the elderly in hospital who are to undergo a general anaesthetic for any operation is described in Chapters 3 and 4 on anaesthesia and the medical problems are dealt with in Chapter 2.

Before operation, however trivial it may be going to be, a careful examination should be made of the patient and the function and state of all systems noted. This must be done even if the patient is to be sent home the same day, after a fracture has been treated, as an outpatient. So often in the old, a trivial injury occurs because of a fall or stumble caused by some other illness, which must be excluded before treatment is given. It is easy to fail to diagnose a very mild stroke in an old lady, brought by ambulance to the accident department, and who has a Colles's fracture. Lying comfortably on the stretcher until the anaesthetic is given and the fracture set and put into a plaster cast the slight signs may be missed and the patient sent home later that day and put straight to bed, from which she may not be able to get up on the next day because of the underlying condition.

The Injury

"What made you fall?". This is a vital question and must be asked of every patient seen. The patient who is active and falls in the street is usually unfortunate enough to have had a true accident; but not always is this so. When she was walking she might have looked up sharply and sustained a drop attack; this may explain her accusation of tripping on an uneven pavement, where no unevenness existed. Perhaps the patient fell in the bus because she was deaf and did not hear the conductor telling her to hold tight. The list of possibilities is long and all aspects of the accident must be investigated very thoroughly.

Those patients who fall at home need even more intensive enquiry to determine the reason for the fall because the prognosis for any patient with a serious fracture which has occurred at home, particularly in the bedroom or kitchen, can be poor. It is possible that the patient did have a proper fall, slipping on unnoticed grease on the kitchen floor, or tripping over a ruckled carpet in the bedroom; but such explanations, freely given by patients to account for the fall, are rarely the truth and the fall occurred for no good reason to be found at the time; later investigation will usually produce evidence that some other concurrent condition was the cause. When an unexplained fall occurs it is often a symptom of the impending dissolution of the patient.

Between these two categories of the active person with a proper accident and the failing, aged patient with no explanation of the fall come a group which cannot be placed accurately on their admission to hospital and this is because they may have lain at home on the floor for some while; they may have hypothermia, they may be very anaemic through the malnutrition so commonly found in the elderly, there may have been a definite illness (such as pneumonia) to cause the fall. These patients are resuscitated as quickly as is reasonably possible so that they may have the fracture fixed the next day. Thereafter patients tend to fall into one or other of the two categories described above. It is quite remarkable how many patients are so much better after the fracture has been fixed and blood loss has been replaced that it is obvious that they are basically in the fit group of patients; others will quite obviously require intensive further general geriatric and orthopaedic rehabilitation preferably in the geriatric orthopaedic unit.

Prevention of Infection at Operation

All geriatric patients with a fracture should have antibiotics exhibited with the premedication and continued for at least a week after operation and if necessary longer, according to the size of procedure done. It is our practice, if the operation is big, such as for a fracture near the hip, to use a cephalosporin, at first by injection (Ceporin) and then by mouth (Ceporex). For the smaller operations flucloxacillin and ampicillin (Magnapen) gives an excellent cover. At operation the wound should be liberally sprinkled with an antibiotic powder and one often used is a mixture of penicillin and streptomycin (Crystamycin). A gramme of this powder sprinkled into a moderate size wound causes no local reaction and appears to be efficacious, but it must be combined with systemic cover.

The routine use of antibiotic cover should never give false confidence. The surgical technique must always be exemplary; slipshod surgery and poor aseptic technique will produce infected wounds. Even with the most admirable attention to detail in the theatre and in doing the operation there is always a high risk of infection in the debilitated geriatric patient and so there should be no hesitation in giving antibiotics at the time of an operation. Further, old people, in one way or another, can contaminate their wounds by incontinence or wandering fingers. The anaesthetist will also often wish to have antibiotic cover for a few days after the operation, particularly in the bronchitic patient and those with other affections of the lungs.

The Prevention of Fractures

The two main causes of severe fractures in the elderly are, first, weakness of the bone from osteoporosis which predisposes to the second cause, a careless step, unguarded movement or fall. There is still no adequate cure for osteoporosis and faith should not be put in prescribing multiple drugs for an old person in the hopes of preserving the strength of the bone, other than those discussed in Chapter 2. However, it is apparent that osteoporosis in most patients is associated with considerable loss of muscular tone and therefore one aid to the prevention of fractures is continued exercise. Whether the loss of muscular tone is purely a physiological attribute of old age or whether it is secondary to some other cause is unknown. Nevertheless it is well recognised that activity is the best method of preventing osteoporosis in a limb that is immobilised in plaster, irrespective of the age of the patient; similarly, the worst place for generalised osteoporosis is in bed, resting. Gravity is eliminated and the normal muscular tone necessary to preserve the erect posture is lost and more osteoporosis is encouraged.

Falls can be prevented; the advice to use a walking stick (or a long handled umbrella when pride prevents the use of the former) may stop falls in the street or garden, especially if there is any tendency to giddiness.

Good eyesight cannot always be maintained, but it must be maintained as best as possible, as must hearing. The elderly must be encouraged to cross busy roads with even more than the usual care; a white stick for the partially sighted is a help.

In the home, a good light over the stairs is essential and must be left on at night, as should one in or near the lavatory. Loose carpets, especially when old, ruckled and worn, must be banned. Other carpets should have no loose edge that might cause a trip, but should be tacked down. A double bannister, one on each side of the stairs, is essential for the infirm person.

Handles to assist in the bath and lavatory can prevent a catastrophe and no bath mat that slips on the floor should be retained; instead a non-slip rubber mat may be used, both in and out of the bath or shower.

Excessive small tables and stools should be put away, they may easily cause a fall. Heavy furniture is often used by old people as support and should be steady and on even feet or casters. Front and back door steps should have a hand rail and there should be a raised shelf on which milk and other deliveries may be put so that, in the morning, they may be taken in easily. An icy step is a veritable death trap to an old person.

Discipline at night when getting out of bed is important. A light must always be used, and a few seconds taken sitting before standing may avoid a fall caused by postural hypertension.

Drop attacks must be guarded against by not looking suddenly upwards or sideways.

Loose flex to a lamp, television or telephone must be reduced to the least possible, but it is important that the telephone should have an extension to the bedside and that, in whatever position it may be, it can be reached from the floor if by chance the old person does fall and cannot get up. Often they can crawl to the telephone to summon aid.

Strong night sedation drugs, particularly the barbiturates, confuse the patient and are a cause of falls and should not be used.

The list is long; commonsense and an understanding of infirmity will dictate the necessary action in any particular case. Even so, too stringent regulations will hamper the enjoyment of life and reduce independence; rather than have the patient adhere to none of the advice it is better to choose the most important items only so that at least these will be accepted.

After Care

The programme for the patient should be produced at the time of operation. It is based on the type of injury and the probable duration of incapacity combined with the general condition of the patient and the circumstances in which she lived. The type of operation done may also have to be considered. The use of suction drains and infusions that continue after operation are no contraindication to early walking. The care of the bladder will be considered, as will the bowels. Other complaints that so often beset the patient may need to be treated.

It is therefore very necessary that all concerned with the treatment of the particular patient should know what is to be done, how soon certain objectives have got to be reached and what the present capabilities of the patient are. This requires intensive teamwork.

Rehabilitation After Operation

The geriatric orthopaedic unit is described in Chapter 14 as well as its methods. However, in the acute orthopaedic wards a similar team is necessary, and will meet at each ward round to discuss each patient. The ward sister, the physiotherapist, the occupational therapist, the medical social worker and the secretary are all necessary for the quick rehabilitation of the geriatric patient whether otherwise fit or ill.

Whether the injury be in the upper or lower limb personal independence is to be achieved first and secondly independence at home. This is true return to function in the elderly. Nothing must stand in the way of these two objectives. Therefore the day after the operation the patient is out of bed and, as soon as possible, is allowed to get dressed. The expression "allowed to get dressed" is used deliberately because for many patients part of the assessment of independence is to see the patient dress. It is very easy, if the patient is being slow to get their clothes on, for a nurse or some other person to start helping; the real disability that, for example, the patient is unable to put on her own underclothes without assistance will pass unnoticed and thus independence is not achieved. Some patients may take up to an hour to get dressed but when this is considered against the background of nothing much else to do all day when they go home, it does not matter. With time there will be an improvement in this performance, particularly once the patient gets home and back to familiar surroundings. Finally, getting dressed is an excellent general exercise.

As soon as the patient is able to be out of bed, usually the day after the operation, then a commode will be used rather than the bedpan and the more the patient has to be in and out of bed the more rehabilitation does this give in itself. The exercise of doing this is considerable. The commode next to the bed is used only until the patient is able to walk to the nearby lavatory; this is the next most important step because, once achieved, the patient may be considered personally independent provided there are no other conditions such as mental confusion or nocturnal incontinence that vitiate it.

At least once each week there will be a formal ward round with the whole team present at which every aspect of the patient will be considered. In the acute orthopaedic ward the main problem is to divide those patients that are able to get home directly, or after some sheltered care with a relative or in a preconvalescent ward, and those who will need further intensive medical and surgical rehabilitation in the geriatric orthopaedic unit. It is the practice at Hastings to allow preconvalescence at five days or so after a fracture has been fixed. To be able to manage the patient must be personally independent and able to walk, with an aid of one or other type, some 15 metres without having to rest sitting down. The speed at which this is done is immaterial.

Pre-Convalescence

It is valuable to have sheltered accommodation available to ease the burden on the acute orthopaedic ward and to which patients may go as soon after operation as they become independent.

Thus the patient who has had a fractured neck of femur replaced by a cemented Thompson prosthesis, and who has been otherwise active and healthy will go to a preconvalescent bed at about the fifth day. The facilities available are full hotel cover, with nursing available but not given normally except in the daily clinic, when wounds will be dressed, stitches removed and drugs given. Other drugs needing repeated dosage are given out at meal times. Supervision is present the whole time but as the patient improves it becomes less and less. In general, the patient is self sufficient each day and at the end of two or three weeks is able to return home to an independent existence.

The Ill Patient

The ill patient who is admitted with a fracture—usually one near the hip—and who was leading a most inactive life before has a bad prognosis which can only be ameliorated by the most intensive rehabilitation after an operation that will have, once and for all, obviated the fracture. At the earliest possible moment the patient will be transferred from the acute orthopaedic ward to the geriatric orthopaedic unit. This is fully described in Chapter 14.

Many patients are admitted from old people's homes, nursing homes, geriatric wards or from one form or another of long stay beds. It is possible, occasionally, to return the patient to a greater level of independence than before the fracture by the treatment of all the ailments that co-existed, but usually, despite intensive efforts, the independence of such a patient is lowered and the prognosis both for mortality in hospital or for return to the previous level of activity is poor. If death does not supervene within a few weeks, the outcome is often admission to a long stay hospital bed. Close co-operation of the geriatric physician with the orthopaedic surgeon is nowhere more important; and that the geriatrician should understand fully that there is no orthopaedic lesion holding the patient in bed or in hospital will be sufficient to have the patient transferred to the proper care of the geriatric department.

References

Gallannaugh, S. C. (1974). Supracondylar fractures of the femur in the elderly: treatment by internal fixation. *Injury, The British Journal of Accident Surgery* **5** No. 3.
Pool, C. J. F. (1973). Colles's fracture. A prospective study of treatment. *Journal of Bone and Joint Surgery* **55B** No. 3.

9

Fractures Near the Hip

C. G. ATTENBOROUGH

Fractures near the hip are of two types. First are those that occur in the femoral neck and are either subcapital or transcervical; second are the trochanteric fractures. Both types may be caused by relatively severe violence but, in the old patient with osteoporotic bones, a subcapital fracture especially may occur with very trivial violence or even none at all. The latter must often be considered as a symptom of the impending dissolution of the patient. There are also those patients with true pathological fractures and, finally, the stress fracture that occurs with little or no warning.

This "disease" of the elderly, as fractures of the neck of the femur should perhaps be called, sometimes achieves epidemic proportions, particularly in areas of the country where there are a large number of retired and old people. Such an epidemic can place a very grave burden on an orthopaedic department which is not geared to cope with this great problem. With proper organisation, however, large numbers of fractures of the neck of the femur can be successfully treated, rehabilitated and sent out of hospital without blocking all the available orthopaedic beds (Devas and D'Arcy, 1976).

Management

It must be emphasised that the treatment of a fracture of the neck of the femur starts as soon as the patient is discovered after the accident. In old patients it is essential to eliminate pressure on the skin from hard surfaces as soon as possible. Sometimes several hours may elapse before the injured patient is discovered and during this time irreparable harm may have been done to the skin because of the patient laying on a hard floor. Pads of thick sponge plastic, carried in the ambulance, are placed under the sacrum and heels as soon as the patient is put on to a stretcher. The pads should remain in position until the patient is again mobile after operation. Nothing predisposes more to bed sores than several hours on a stretcher in the ambulance and in the accident department, later on the x-ray table and later still on a hard operation table. There is no difficulty in the radiography or in operating on the patients with the pads in place. It is possible that a greater use of water beds whilst the patient is awaiting operation might also help to reduce the incidence of pressure sores.

As soon as the patient is admitted a full examination must be carried out. It is usual to discover several other conditions apart from the fractures and immediate treatment may be required for some. Diabetes and cardiac failure are amongst the most common. A check is made for hypothermia and the haemoglobin, blood group and electrolytes are estimated. Two units of blood are cross matched. Although it is perhaps preferable in most instances to operate as soon as possible, some patients are dehydrated and a delay of a few hours, even up to 24 and, rarely, 48 hours, is permissible while the dehydration and any electrolyte imbalance are corrected. Patients already in heart failure may require to be given digoxin before operation, and diabetes must be stabilised.

It is our practice to operate at the next available operating session providing that the general physical state is considered to be as good as it ever will be. This is usually the day after admission. If the patient is in pain while awaiting surgery, then light skin traction is applied using the "Ventafoam" type of traction and not an adhesive type of strapping, to avoid injury to the skin.

Infection after operation is a most important cause of morbidity. It may involve the wound, the lungs or the genito urinary system. In the wound there must also be added to the normal hazard of operation the wandering fingers of the elderly confused patient disturbing the dressing and thus causing a direct infection of the incision. Breathing exercises are started before operation and continued afterwards. Even if continent before the fall, many female patients will be incontinent of urine after a fracture of the femoral neck and in these, the immediate use of an indwelling catheter may help to prevent a sacral pressure sore. An antibiotic is given until after the catheter is removed and we prefer a broad spectrum antibiotic such as Septrin.

Because of the dangers of wound and chest infection, it is our practice to use an antibiotic cover for the operation and, in most instances, Magnapen is given in a dose of 500 milligrams four times a day. Before operation the first dose is given intramuscularly with the premedication and further intramuscular injections are given until the patient can take the capsules easily by mouth. This is continued for at least a week after the operation and, as Devas and D'Arcy have shown in their review of subcapital fractures (1976) wound infection can be kept below 5% but chest infection still occurred in 10% of the 161 patients reviewed.

The treatment of this disease of the elderly must, therefore, be seen as a treatment of the whole patient and any operation is considered to be but an incident in the whole process of rehabilitating the patient to the condition before operation, sometimes with the bonus of some chronic condition such as pernicious anaemia having been diagnosed and treated. With this in mind it must be emphasised that any operation must leave the patient without a fracture so that, apart from attention to the wound, no further treatment is needed so that the rehabilitation of the patient as a whole may continue forthwith.

The division of the fractures into subcapital and trochanteric is only of importance because of the different aetiology and the different surgical technique. Thereafter progress should be the same (Fig. 1).

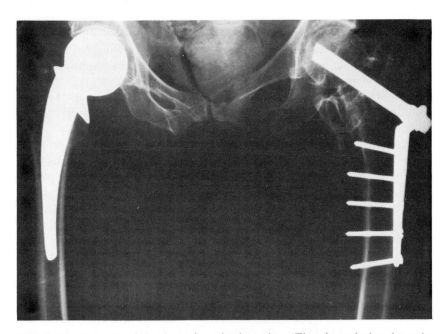

FIG. 1 The hallmark of the decrepit geriatric patient. The pin and plate kept the patient in hospital for eight days; four years later she took four weeks to rehabilitate and return home after the replacement of the femoral head with the Thompson prosthesis.

Subcapital Fractures

The controversy in many centres still continues between those who advocate the treatment by internal fixation and those who prefer replacement. When Smith Petersen first introduced his method of internal fixation of fractures of the neck of the femur with a trifin nail, it was a tremendous advance in the treatment of this difficult condition. The use of internal fixation in various forms has continued ever since and, if it were always successful, it would undoubtedly be preferable to a replacement operation. The method, however, fails in some 30% of patients and this means a second operation or considerable morbidity in one patient in every three; further, the older the patient the higher the incidence of failure becomes.

The increased time in bed and in hospital because of a method of fracture fixation of the femoral neck that fails or cannot be trusted for immediate weightbearing results in delay in the rehabilitation programme and often permanent loss of function and, as a result, loss of independence.

Internal fixation probably fails for one of three reasons. First, the fracture may fail to unite; second, the fracture unites and avascular necrosis of the head develops, leading to collapse of the hip joint; third, the fracture may unite and, at a later date, give rise to osteoarthritis without avascular necrosis apparently supervening.

There are many reasons why the fracture may fail to unite but failure of fixation by single or multiple pinning of a severely osteoporotic bone is probably the most important. If the head of the femur is very soft then, no matter how well the fracture is reduced and how well placed the internal fixation, cutting out of the nail is going to lead to a failure of the fracture to unite.

Avascular necrosis of the head of the femur is most common when there has been wide separation of the fragments but it is by no means unknown without any displacement, particularly after the insertion of a trifin nail.

The development of osteoarthritis without avascular necrosis supervening is more common in the active group of patients and may be related to damage to the articular cartilage by the relatively greater violence of the fall in these individuals.

Replacement of the femoral head with a prosthesis eliminates failure from non-union and from avascular necrosis. The mortality rate after operation is no higher than with internal fixation by pinning.

The most important cause of erosion of the acetabular cartilage is the violence which accompanied the fall which produced the injury. This has been emphasised by Devas and D'Arcy (1976) who showed that, if replacement of the femoral head is used as a treatment in fractures of the neck of the femur under the age of 60, 43% developed acetabular erosion. Between the ages of 60 and 69, 22% developed this erosion. Between the ages of 70 and 79 the percentage fell to 14% and over 80 to 1.7%. Occasionally pain may arise after the replacement of the femoral head by a prosthesis, usually from erosion of the acetabular articular cartilage.

Erosion may also be caused by inserting a prosthesis which is too small, producing central damage to the cartilage from point bearing of a small head in a larger acetabulum. It is possible that, in some instances, too large a prosthesis, which does not fit snugly into the acetabulum may produce a ring of peripheral damage to the cartilage. It must be emphasised that only some of the patients with acetabular erosion have symptoms that need further treatment but in view of these figures, a replacement operation as the treatment for subcapital fractures of the neck of the femur should probably be confined to the elderly patient, with an apparent age of 70 or more. At Hastings it is believed that, in this age group, elimination of non-union and avascular necrosis and the rapid return of function far outweigh the disadvantages. In younger patients, under the age of 70, internal fixation may be preferable and a second operation on such patients may often be needed if complications supervene. There may even be a place for total hip replacement in younger patients in whom it is known that the violence has been sufficient to disrupt the fragments widely or to damage severely the acetabular cartilage.

At any age group there may be some patients in whom a second operation will be required for acetabular erosion after femoral head replacement for a subcapital fracture. Such an operation will be made much easier when the techniques for the initial operation devised by Monk and more recently by Devas become more widely used. These techniques use a femoral head which will fit the acetabular component of a total hip replacement. This head fits into a cup which is the correct size to fit the acetabulum and is not, of course, cemented. In the case of the Devas type the metal head of the femur articulates with a high density polyethylene insert in a metal acetabular cup, of which there are sizes to fit any dimension of the patient's acetabulum. When completed movement occurs both between the acetabulum and the cup and between the femoral head and the high density polyethylene insert within the cup. If a second operation is required because of acetabular erosion, the acetabular component is removed and replaced by a cemented acetabular component which fits the femoral head already in position and avoids the necessity of further reaming and recementing of a prosthesis in the femoral medullary cavity.

These newer implants may come into routine use but at present at Hastings, patients over the age of 70 are treated by the removal of the femoral head and the insertion of a Thompson prosthesis cemented into the medullary cavity of the femur. We believe the benefits of almost immediate relief of pain and increased confidence when weightbearing is commenced, far outweigh the possible complications of the use of cement. The Austin Moore prosthesis has been used at times but it has not been found so satisfactory first, because it is more difficult to insert through a relatively small exposure, and second because it did not give the same confidence to the patient on immediate walking the day after operation.

OPERATIVE TECHNIQUE USING A THOMPSON PROSTHESIS

At Hastings the antero-lateral approach as described by McKee and Watson Farrar (1966) is used in all cases of replacement of the femoral head for fractured neck of the femur. We have found that the use of the common posterior approach has led to a substantial number of dislocations. Despite early mobilisation, the use of the antero-lateral approach has reduced the dislocation rate to 2%.

The patient is placed either in the supine or in the lateral position. An incision is made from the antero-superior iliac spine to the posterior aspect of the greater trochanter and then down the outer side of the femur for a short distance. The deep fascia is divided and the capsule of the hip is exposed by separating the rectus femoris muscle in front from the gluteus medius behind. Several large vessels need to be coagulated while deepening the incision. A longitudinal incision is made in the anterior capsule of the hip joint from the rim of the acetabulum to the base of the neck of the femur. If the femoral head is large, a cruciate incision in the anterior capsule is sometimes helpful. The femoral head is removed with a corkscrew-like extractor and this is sometimes made easier by placing a bone lever within the acetabulum. Care must be taken, however, to avoid damage to the articular cartilage of the acetabulum.

The stump of the femoral neck is trimmed and often a centimetre or more of bone needs to be removed from the calcar femorale, in order to permit final reduction of the new head into the acetabulum.

It is very important to estimate accurately the size of the Thompson prosthesis to be used. The femoral head is measured with a caliper and the appropriate size of prosthesis is then inserted into the acetabulum as a trial. If it is too small, it will enter and leave the acetabulum easily. If it is too large, it is also easy to remove. The correct size is the one in which insertion of the head is relatively easy but extraction is difficult because of the vacuum caused by the close fit.

The leg is now externally rotated and adducted so that the medullary cavity of the femur can be reached. The femoral broach is tapped gently into the femur and it is of great importance that it is running within the medullary cavity. In elderly osteoporotic patients it is all too easy to perforate the posterior lateral cortex of the femur. A trial fit is now carried out, inserting the stem of the Thompson prosthesis into the medullary cavity of the femur and also estimating the degree of difficulty of reduction of the head into the acetabulum. If it appears that reduction will be very difficult, then a further small amount of bone length may be removed from the femoral neck.

A catheter is placed in the medullary cavity of the femur and attached to a sucker. If the catheter is found to suck blood and fat, then it is almost certainly within the medullary cavity. If the catheter fails to suck blood or fat, then there is a distinct possibility that it has passed through a hole in the postero-lateral cortex of the femur and the medullary cavity should be carefully probed to find out if a false passage has been made. If necessary, the femoral broach can be used once again to correct this error.

Cement is gently pushed into the medullary cavity. The use of the catheter and sucker in an elderly patient will reduce the pressure within the medullary cavity. It is possible that this may help to prevent either fat or the cement monomer entering the circulation which, if it occurs, can cause the sudden collapse of the patient at or just after the insertion of the cement.

The Thompson prosthesis is pushed gently into the cement in the medullary cavity and, once the cement is hard, is reduced into the acetabulum. In some instances it may be felt advisable to instil a local antibiotic into the wound, before closing it in the usual way using suction drainage.

Trochanteric Fractures

Once again it should be emphasised that, in the treatment of a geriatric patient after an injury, the fracture should be eliminated so that rapid rehabilitation is not impeded. There is no place for the treatment of trochanteric fractures in the elderly by immobilisation in bed on traction. It is probable that nearly all these fractures will unite on traction without operation but few will require less than eight weeks in bed and the delay in recovery of function may well lead to bedsores, to loss of independence and even death.

TECHNIQUE OF OPERATION

It is our practice to use a McLaughlin pin and plate. One piece nail plates are rather more difficult to insert with speed. If the fracture is to be eliminated and the patient allowed to start weightbearing immediately after operation it is essential that the pin and plate should be accurately placed. In the soft bone of a geriatric patient a too oblique position in the neck of the femur may cause penetration of the nail into the hip joint on weightbearing. It is, therefore, advisable to use a more transversely placed nail. In some very ill patients internal fixation may be life-saving and, if necessary, the operating time can be shortened by dispensing with radiographs and placing the guide wire by feel alone. It should always be possible to insert a nail in an acceptable position. The details of the operation are otherwise as normally done.

Care After Operation

The care of patients who have been treated by a cemented Thompson prosthesis for a subcapital fracture or a pin and plate for a trochanteric fracture is very much the same because in both the fracture has been eliminated.

During and after the operation most patients require two pints of blood. Intravenous fluids are then continued for at least 48 hours after operation. These patients are often poor drinkers with a poor urinary output unless intravenous fluids are continued. It is also helpful to keep the intravenous drip running in case of a sudden collapse. At the end of 48 hours, the electrolytes and haemoglobin are re-assessed and, if satisfactory, the intravenous drip is discontinued. The suction drainage is usually removed at 48 hours unless drainage continues freely.

The patient must be out of bed on the day after operation and sits in a chair for up to two hours and stands and walks. Thereafter they walk with the physiotherapist at least twice a day and as soon as they are able are encouraged to walk as far as the toilet. The time of sitting in a chair is gradually increased to four hours. The theoretical objection to patients sitting are not applicable to geriatric patients, for whom sitting is normal for many hours of the day, whereas in younger adults a more active life is normal and it is in these patients that a long period of sitting after an operation may predispose to phlebothrombosis. One advantage of early walking is an increase in confidence and, because of this, the patients move more when they are in bed and again this helps to avoid phlebothrombosis and pressure sores.

Throughout this period it is essential to continue regular skin care of all possible pressure areas until the patient is out of bed most of the time. The type of skin care varies from hospital to hospital but essentially it should consist of circular massage of the potential pressure area with soap and water for at least two minutes. The area is then thoroughly rinsed, dried and powdered. In cases where there is any sign of redness, instead of powdering, the area should be massaged once again with a mixture of 50% oil and surgical spirit.

A radiograph is usually taken on the day after operation but, because the surgeon will already be satisfied that he has eliminated the fracture at the time of operation, the patient should not be delayed from weightbearing for the result. Sutures are removed at 12 to 14 days. It is not necessary to keep the patient in hospital for this, and many patients go home or to a convalescent home four to five days after operation. In those patients in whom supervised rehabilitation will be necessary for a longer period or where pre-existing conditions require further medical treatment transfer to the geriatric orthopaedic unit is arranged within a few days of operation.

Complications

Infection has already been mentioned. Deep vein thrombosis is the other complication of the operation itself and occurs in only 5% of patients.

The remaining complications of the treatment of the neck of the femur in geriatric patients are mainly those one would expect in any group of elderly patients and are due to the associated diseases from which these patients suffered before the fracture of the neck of the femur occurred. Providing that the surgeon eliminates the fracture and there is no infection and providing that pressure sores are avoided, then it will only be the other pre-existing conditions that will delay the return of the patient to full function and independence.

Fractures of the Acetabulum

Fractures involving the acetabulum should be treated symptomatically providing that they are slight, as they usually are. The patient can usually be mobilised and at least partially weightbearing within two to three weeks. The more severe fractures of the acetabulum, and central dislocations of the hip, are not common in the elderly but, when they do occur they cause considerable difficulty.

Traction may have to be used to control pain, and if it has to be continued for a few weeks it will, of necessity, considerably delay the return to independence. Time on traction should be kept to the shortest possible, being set symptomatically rather than by radiographs. The patient should be allowed to sit out of bed as soon as the pain will allow but full weightbearing will usually have to be delayed for six to eight weeks. In some instances an early total hip replacement may be considered, possibly using an acetabular component with a rim to abut against the margin of the acetabulum.

References

Devas, M. B. and D'Arcy, J. (1976). Treatment of fractures of the femoral neck by replacement with the Thompson prosthesis. *Journal of Bone and Joint Surgery* **54B.**

McKee, G. K. and Watson-Farrar, J. (1966). Replacement of arthritic hips by the Watson-Farrar prosthesis. *Journal of Bone and Joint Surgery* **48B,** 245.

10

Fractures in the Elderly—
General Considerations

MICHAEL DEVAS

Fractures of the Lower Limb

The management of fractures of the femur near the hip has been dealt with in Chapter 9; it is the key to the treatment of all other fractures in the elderly, which is to obviate the fracture in such a way that function and independence are at once restored. Once this principle is understood there will on the whole be no great problems encountered, although there will be, on occasion, a time when the resources of surgery fail, and no formal orthopaedic procedure is possible. Nevertheless, the principles behind any surgery undertaken must always be adhered to rigidly and, in this way, the early rehabilitation of the patient will lead to a quick return to the activities of daily living and a satisfactory quality of life.

FRACTURES OF THE UPPER FEMORAL SHAFT

Pin and plate fixation for trochanteric fractures is so successful that the same method is used for fractures high in the femoral shaft. The only difference is the length of the plate which must be long enough to allow four, or more, screws to be put in distal to the fracture. The fracture in this part of the femur is often caused by considerable violence, such as falling downstairs or off a chair while hanging up curtains, and may have one or more extensions going upwards towards the trochanters which jeopardise the grip of the screws above the site of the obvious fracture. For this reason the pin attached to the plate is necessary, transferring the strain to the uninjured femoral neck. The fine lines of the fracture extension upwards can well be missed in emergency radiographs and, for the same reason, intramedullary fixation may be disastrous with separation of the proximal femur into fragments.

A seven-hole pin and plate will be satisfactory for a low trochanteric fracture, that is one at or just below the level of the lesser trochanter, provided four screws grip the bone firmly in the distal fragment. Less than four screws will jeopardise the safety of walking the patient next day. If the fracture is lower than this, then a longer plate must be used. The operation is done in exactly the same way as described for the ordinary pin and plate procedure with a distal extension of the incision.

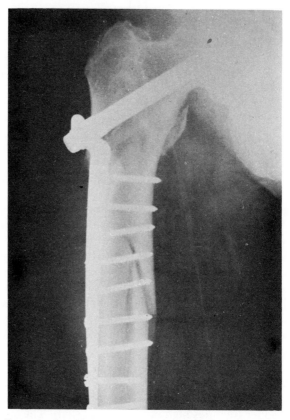

FIG. 1 The radiograph of an 80 year old man who had fallen and fractured the upper third of the shaft of his right femur, which was treated by a pin and a 12 hole plate. He took six weeks to rehabilitate but was then able to go home to an independent existence.

There must be no rule of thumb about the number of screws that will be satisfactory below the fracture, but the patient as a whole, and the grip of the screws in the bone in particular, must always be assessed and necessary allowances made (Fig. 1).

Patients respond well to this procedure and the long incision heals very quickly and without serious morbidity. Because it is in the lateral part of the thigh and the tensor fasciae latae is split to gain access to the underlying vastus lateralis, which is also split, the effect on the quadriceps mechanism as a whole is not serious and the patient may walk the day after the operation.

With the exposure it is important to use two suction drains, one deep and one superficial to the fascia lata; the posterior and lateral aspects of the thigh usually have much adipose tissue only loosely attached to the underlying fascia and haematoma formation can occur very easily without proper drainage, and once the patient is up, may track down the thigh. Therefore the superficial drain must be put in with care to drain the most distal part of the wound.

The grip of plates with seven or more holes is usually good but if the bone is very osteoporotic the grip, even when using a tap with non-selftapping screws, will be greatly increased by using high density polythene plates.

The geriatric patient is safe to walk on this type of fixation whereas, in the younger person, the muscle strength and the walking ability will be too great for the strength of the plate which may bend, break, or become loose; this does not occur in the older patient.

FRACTURES OF THE CENTRE AND LOWER SHAFT OF THE FEMUR

The fractured shaft of femur in an old person must be treated as an emergency, just as a fracture near the hip, and operation done as soon as possible. The loss of blood and the shock occasioned by this injury is greater than that caused by a fracture near the hip. Pain is considerable, and old people do not stand such pain well; heavy sedation to alleviate the pain carries its own problems in an old person and must be used with great care. Because of the pain, and because of all the same reasons that apply to the fracture near the hip, the patient should be operated upon as soon as is practical, that is, within 24 hours, and intramedullary fixation done.

The patient, prepared in the usual way for the operation, is placed on the theatre table with the knees bent over the end and the head of the table tilted downwards. This will give gentle traction against the calves. The limb is then cleansed and towelled.

The intramedullary nail is inserted through the knee. A small incision is made, usually on the medial side of the patellar tendon, but according to the shape of the knee and any deformities that are present it may be made on the lateral side of the tendon. The latter, and the patella, are then retracted. It is often helpful to straighten the knee slightly to release the tension of the quadriceps expansion and so assist in allowing the patella and its tendon to move aside.

The synovia is entered and the intercondylar notch exposed. Using a small osteotome or gouge a hole is made so that it will lie not only centrally in the notch but also centrally in relation to the anterior and posterior cortices of the femoral shaft. A small amount of cancellous bone is scooped out around the edge of the hole to make a shelf which will be used later.

A measured guidewire is inserted into the lower femoral shaft and by using simple traction and gentle manipulation of the thigh it is often possible to slide the guidewire into the upper fragment even without an image intensifier. If this proves impossible or time consuming a small incision is made directly anterior to the fracture and deepened through the quadriceps muscle, the

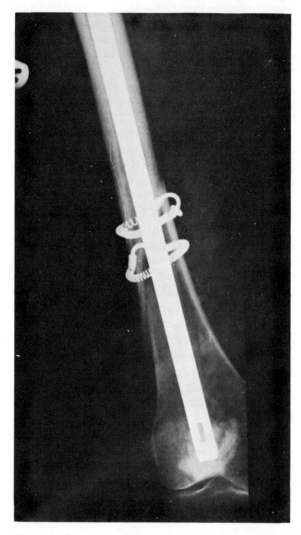

FIG. 2 The radiograph of a woman of 77 who had injured her right leg. A Küntscher nail was inserted through the knee and two Attenborough springs were placed round the fracture itself. Both the incisions were small and the patient did well. The cement in the lower femur can be seen.

fibres of which are gently separated until one or two fingers can feel the bone ends. It is then possible to manipulate the fracture. Often failure to have done so by the earlier blind attempt is because there has been muscle interposition, preventing proper reduction. The guidewire is then passed into the upper fragment and check radiographs taken. An intramedullary nail of suitable length and diameter is inserted over the guidewire and driven home with particular care to make sure that rotation is correctly maintained.

If the nail then shows that it has gripped both top and bottom fragments very firmly some cement is mixed and packed into the hole in the inter-condylar notch and forms a satisfactory plug, resting distally on the recess scooped out earlier. This not only prevents the intramedullary nail from slipping down into the knee joint but also acts as a cork, preventing an influx of marrow tissue, fat, blood and cancellous bone fragments into the knee (Fig. 2).

If cement is not available it is best to make the hole into the intercondylar notch slightly rectangular rather than square and then the rectangle of bone removed can be replaced after the nail has been inserted, but pushed more deeply and then turned through 90 degrees so that the long axis of the rectangular piece of bone lies across the short axis of the hole. This will prevent the nail sliding distally, but will not prevent seepage. It is necessary then to use a suction drain in the knee. This need not be done if the hole in the lower femur has been plugged with cement.

After this operation the patient may walk the next day.

Occasionally, and particularly if the fracture is a little low down the shaft, the lower fragment has a much larger intramedullary cavity than that in the shaft above, and does not fix the lower fragment firmly. Reaming the upper shaft is of little avail in osteoporotic bone. To correct instability of the nail in the lower fragment, the stacking technique is used. A short, large diameter nail is selected and slid home, stacked, or locked, into the open channel of the other nail already in place. A satisfactory fixation is then obtained for the lower fragment.

SUPRACONDYLAR FRACTURES OF THE FEMUR

This fracture occurs in the very old and it is the experience at Hastings that often such a patient has already had previous operations to deal with fractures near the hip. The supracondylar fracture of the femur, more often than not, involves the knee joint by a vertical component of the fracture passing between the condyles. This can be difficult to overcome and a special plate has been devised to control the whole fracture. It is a nail plate which is fixed to the lateral aspect of the lower femur with the nail passing into the lateral condyle. The centre of the nail is cannulated and threaded to take a compression bolt inserted from the medial side.

The patient is prepared for operation in the usual way and, on an ordinary operation table tilted to the good side, a lateral incision is made over the lower third of the thigh extending down to the level of the knee. The fracture is approached and reduced as best possible. Often it is found to be far worse than the radiological assessment, with much comminution.

The guide wire is inserted into the lateral condyle, passed through the medial condyle and penetrates through the skin on the medial side. The position is confirmed radiographically. A cannulated drill may be necessary to make the passage of the nail easier, especially in badly comminuted fractures, but it must not be so large that the fins of the nail do not obtain a good grip. The nail plate is then passed over the guide wire and gently tapped home, using firm support on the medial condyle to prevent undue separation. Once the nail is in place a small incision is made over the guide

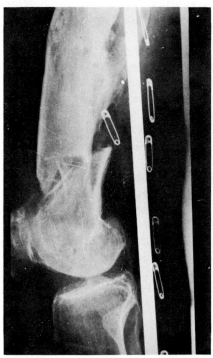 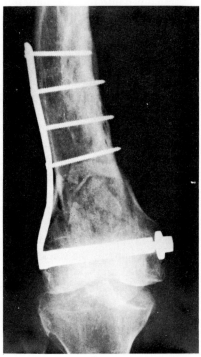

Fig. 3   Fig. 4

FIGS. 3 and 4 An elderly man was involved in a road accident. Previously he had had a compound fracture of his right femur. The radiograph in figure 3 shows that he had sustained a T-shaped fracture of the lower end of the femur, which was treated with a Devas pin and plate, and a reasonable position was obtained. In the radiograph in figure 4 reduction is satisfactory and the fracture between the condyles can be seen.

wire on the medial side of the knee and deepened down to bone. The cannulated bolt is placed over the guide wire and tapped gently into the bone until it engages the central threaded channel of the nail; it may then be screwed in to compress the condyles. The bolt has a large flat head so that it does not cut into osteoporotic bone. The plate is then fixed to the femur with screws. Often the fixation needs a high density polythene plate on the medial side because, even if the screw holes are properly tapped, osteoporosis is so severe that the grip is unsatisfactory (Figs 3 to 5).

The wound is closed with suction drainage; one drain should be left in the knee joint if it has been involved by the fracture as well as one in the lateral wound, and a firm pressure dressing put on. The patient is allowed out of bed to stand and bear weight the next day; once the drainage has ceased the pressure dressing is removed and gentle knee exercises started. Having ensured a reasonable position of the apparatus clinically it is best to pay little heed to the radiographs after operation because the fragmentation that is so often present might appear to contra-indicate early movement and early weightbearing. This must not be the case because, as in the fracture of the elbow which is treated as "a bag of bones", early movement will obtain the best result. Pain is no more severe after this operation than it is for a hip replacement and is controlled as usual. It is quite remarkable that, even if the fragments were not accurately fitted together, nearly painless movement and good walking is achieved. It is very important not to use plaster fixation and equally important to get the patient out of bed the following day.

FRACTURES OF THE PATELLA

A crack fracture of the patella will occur in an old person without very much force; often there will be found no separation of the fragments. A simple test will decide whether the patient needs immobilisation in a plaster cylinder or not; if straight leg raising is possible when the patient is first seen then there is every indication to allow the patient to continue walking, but with the knee firmly supported in a crepe bandage, which can be applied over cotton wool. If movement is still painful, the bandaging should be extended from ankle to thigh and over this a very light "eggshell" plaster cast is applied. Although the plaster cast may crack it will still prevent movement sufficient to cause pain and, being very light, will not hamper the patient to any great extent but will allow her to continue with an independent existence. Care should be taken when applying the compression bandage that it is not so tight that it causes swelling of the foot; a useful precaution is always to provide a Tubigrip support from the toes to the lower edge of the pressure dressing or bandage.

The stellate fracture of the patella is not common, but it should, as in other ages, be excised. It is best to do this through a lateral incision and to enter the knee joint through the capsule and then to enucleate the fragments rather than to approach the patella anteriorly; the quadriceps expansion lying on the medial side of the patella and that part which passes superficial to the patella is left intact; further, the wound in the lateral expansion, lying as it does in the direction of its fibres, is not strained by the contracting quadriceps in straight leg raising. It will be found that the patient, having the usual pressure dressing, will be able to raise the straight leg after the operation and once this is achieved walking may be started.

The transverse fracture with displacement should be fixed. A useful method is to use a bolt with two washers (or an ordinary screw with two small high density polythene plates is satisfactory) to hold the fragments together. The tear in the lateral expansion is sewn up in the usual way, a pressure dressing applied and the patient may be up and walking the following day.

In the elderly there are fractures of the patella which, although not a single undisplaced crack and which have more than two fragments, do not have to be excised and will heal with the same ease as the undisplaced crack fracture. It is always worth trying conservative treatment because it will lose no time.

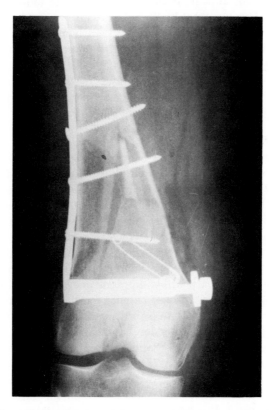

FIG. 5 A radiograph showing a satisfactory compression plating for a very comminuted and (originally) displaced fracture of the lower end of the femur which extended into the intercondylar notch.

FRACTURES OF THE TIBIAL PLATEAU

The varying degrees of severity of the fractures that occur at the upper tibial plateau call for a meticulous form of internal fixation, usually using bolts with washers. This can be so secure in an old person that walking with full weightbearing may be allowed. Should this not seem safe, a light plaster cylinder may be applied (Figs 6 and 7).

Displacement must be corrected, and damaged menisci removed, as in the younger patient.

FRACTURES OF THE UPPER TIBIA

The high fracture of the tibia just below the tibial plateau at about the level of the tibial tubercle is difficult to treat because it is not easy to get a firm plate fixation above the fracture. Often there is no treatment available

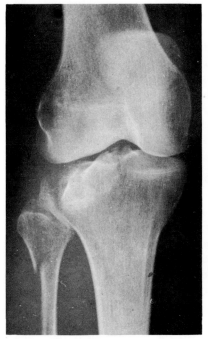
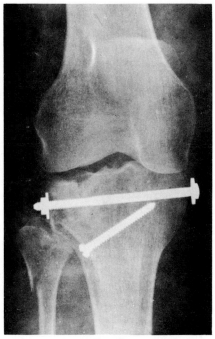

Fig. 6   Fig. 7

FIGS. 6 and 7 Radiographs showing the treatment of a fracture of the lateral tibial condyle. Note that the head of the fibula has also been broken. The fracture was elevated and held with a bolt and the lower fragment was screwed back into place. The patient was able to get up at once and to start active knee movements. High density polythene washers have superseded the metal washers because compression is then dynamic and will continue for several weeks.

other than to reduce the fracture and to apply a plaster cylinder. The fracture at that level is often transverse, and early walking may be tried. At the worst the patient can be up partially weightbearing.

FRACTURES OF THE TIBIAL SHAFT

Internal fixation of tibial fractures can be done in much the same way as at any other age group but one fairly simple way of treating a transverse fracture, which is not uncommon in the very old, is to fix it with an intramedullary nail. The approach is from the tibial plateau and special nails need not be used. Through a small incision medial to the patellar ligament the area of bone just behind the patellar tendon is exposed without entering the synovial membrane. A hole is made in the anterior part of the tibial plateau and a guide wire passed down the tibia. It is very unusual to have to open the fracture site to obtain reduction. It must be recognised that the upper two or three inches of the tibial shaft are angulated on the lower shaft so that the anterior edge of the tibial plateau lies directly above the medulla of the central tibial shaft. In this way an ordinary straight intramedullary nail can be passed down the tibia to obtain good fixation. Again, in the old person often osteoporosis has hollowed out the medullary cavity so that it tends to be larger than might be expected; if, despite care, the nail is too small to give adequate stability a further nail may be stacked and driven home to obtain stability, as described for the fracture of the femoral shaft. A pressure dressing is applied from the toes to above knee and the patient allowed up forthwith.

FRACTURES OF THE LOWERMOST THIRD OF THE TIBIA

Occurring, as they often do, in the very old and osteoporotic patient, fractures in the lowest third of the tibia may be very difficult to treat because there is insufficient bone below the fracture to grip either a plate or an intramedullary nail, and yet displacement will occur if the patient is allowed to walk in a plaster cast. Failure to achieve absolute surgical fixation must be accepted but some form of fixation used to hold the position of the fracture and the use of a plaster cast is the best compromise provided the patient is got up and is as active as possible.

This fracture exemplifies a failure of orthopaedic technique. The osteoporotic bone of the very old person does not lend itself to the various procedures that can be done on the younger patient; nor is bed rest to be accepted in the elderly. The solution is yet to be found.

FRACTURES NEAR THE ANKLE

Like all fractures in the elderly these require the general assessment of the patient. If the old person is otherwise hale and hearty, has had a true accident and could apparently manage the ordinary form of below knee walking plaster cast, then this treatment is indicated, if necessary after a manipulation. However, if the patient is obviously very frail then it is wise not to use a plaster cast because almost invariably it will mean the admission of the patient to hospital for a long time because she will not be able to manage an independent existence at home. Therefore an alternative method of treatment is indicated; internal fixation should be done even if it is only for a mild injury. A lateral or medial malleolus alone that is broken and that denies the patient independence should be internally fixed by a screw or screws so that no plaster cast is needed. The worse the fracture the more imperative becomes internal fixation which will vary according to the type of

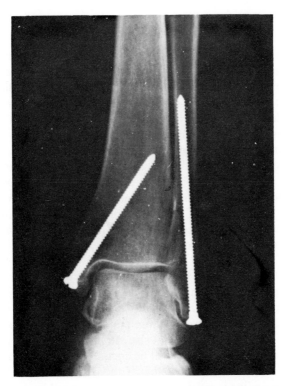

FIG. 8 The radiograph of the ankle of an 89 year old lady who had fallen and sustained a simple Pott's fracture. She had a history of angina and, three days before being admitted, had had a stroke. The day after admission the patient was treated by screw fixation. Satisfactory fixation will allow such patients to do without plaster casts.

fracture. An ordinary long screw passed up from the lateral malleolus into the fibular shaft will control the lateral malleolar fractures but, if the bone is very osteoporotic, a small high density polythene plate will prevent the head of the screw sinking in to the tip of the malleolus. The medial malleolus may be dealt with in much the same way and posterior malleolar fractures should also be screwed home (Fig. 8).

Diastasis of the inferior tibio-fibular joint is rare in the elderly but when it does occur it should be dealt with by a compression screw; the fibula should be over drilled in the usual way so that there can be movement around the screw, while still holding the two bones in apposition. This will prevent pain later and the necessity of removing the screw, as well as allowing painless movement of the ankle in the early stages. No plaster should be used provided the surgeon is able to guarantee that his surgical procedure is secure.

Fractures in the Foot

The elderly, in the ordinary course of life, will either sustain a severe injury to the hindfoot or suffer trivial fractures. Most of the latter are easily dealt with by strapping or pressure dressings but fractures in the hindfoot are often so painful that the part must be rested; this must not stop the patient walking as best possible, using crutches or a frame. During this period it is best not to use plaster casts but firm compression bandages, which are much lighter and which can be removed for active movements and other treatment to reduce swelling. When the patient is at rest, the leg must be elevated.

Usually the severe fracture is in the calcaneum with involvement of the talus and cuboid bone, and the injury occurs in patients who are active; because this is so they are able to manage, once pain and swelling have been controlled, in a light below knee plaster cast with a light plaster boot which is preferable to a rocker or a heel.

FRACTURES OF THE METATARSAL BONES

Lack of insight into the character of a patient may make a metatarsal fracture become a problem unnecessarily. The foot should be firmly bound (this must be done by the surgeon himself and cannot be delegated) and the position explained to the patient that she will have pain and discomfort, but that, if it cannot be tolerated, she will be encumbered with a walking plaster cast. It is explained to the patient that if the discomfort can be borne the method of firm binding is satisfactory, that the bone will heal and that it will heal just as quickly as it would with a plaster cast. However the patient is told also that if she cannot tolerate the pain then a plaster cast will be put on. This reassurance is sufficient usually to allow the patient to accept independence with some pain rather than the restriction of activity. A walking frame for the first week or two is helpful. The best method of firm binding of the foot is with elastic adhesive bandages, which should be put on directly to the skin with no intermediary gauze or padding. If the metatarsal fracture is lateral, then the strapping is applied as a figure of eight starting on the dorsum of the foot, passing medially and under the forefoot to come up from the lateral border of the foot to sweep medially and around the ankle. Each turn follows the previous layer with one or two centimetres of the previous turn of bandage exposed. In this way the lateral border of the foot is lifted and weightbearing made easy. For comfort the adhesive bandage should extend up to the centre of the calf. For fractures of the medial metatarsal bones the direction of bandaging is reversed, to lift the medial side of the foot. Provided the adhesive bandage is retained for three weeks or so, there is little problem about its removal because the natural growth of the epidermis, and the lack of hair in the elderly, allow it to be taken off like a gaiter after cutting the bandage down the front.

This treatment applies to the avulsion fracture of the base of the fifth metatarsal bone which can be very painful but which is in itself a trivial injury. A plaster cast should never be the first treatment and must be kept in reserve for the very few patients who cannot tolerate slight pain or adhesive bandages.

Fractures in the Trunk

The important fractures that occur are those of the vertebral bodies and of the pelvis.

FRACTURES OF THE SPINE

It is difficult at times to distinguish between an osteoporotic fracture of the spine and a compression fracture that has been caused by an accident. The patient may have sat down rather heavily and developed an immediate pain in the back, but there is no radiological difference between an osteoporotic spine that has compressed on its own and one that has been compressed by some injury.

The pain may be very severe and on examination the patient is frightened, anxious, miserable and, because of the inability to move without causing pain, often in great discomfort from a full bladder.

The patient is assessed in the usual way and radiographs obtained.

The essential part of the treatment of this particular fracture is a carefully worded explanation of the condition to the patient, which is adjusted according to intelligence and comprehension. The patient is told that she has severe bruising of a bone in her back and that this is always very painful but that the pain will soon be better; further it is in the best interest of the patient to be moving about as much as possible. It is important not to mention to the patient that she has, in fact, broken her back because nothing detracts more from morale and the idea of getting well quickly than to be told that there exists in oneself a condition for which one was brought up to believe there was little or no possibility of cure. It must be remembered that an octogenarian was born before the beginning of this century when ideas of injury and disease were greatly different from what they are now.

The patient is made comfortable in bed and one pillow given. Provided the one pillow is accepted and is comfortable a second may be added and then a third as time goes by. This is continued until within quite a short time the patient is sitting practically upright. The pain will still be present and may be controlled by mild analgesic drugs but if it requires morphine derivatives to control it then the pace of sitting up should be reduced and a little more rest given.

It is usual to have the patient sitting up in bed within two or three days of admission and as soon as this is achieved there is no difference between sitting on the bed and sitting out of the bed. Again, once sitting on a chair has been accepted the patient is allowed to stand and walk. With continued reassurance by the therapists and nurses and the repeated statement that it is known it is a painful lesion but that it will get better and that the best treatment is to keep moving, the complications of lying immobile on the back on a hard mattress are avoided and the patient can return home very quickly. Mild analgesics must be given; but, again, if opiates are necessary to control pain it is an indication that the pace of rehabilitation is too fast.

The treatment is greatly assisted if a ready made corset is available. Made with firm steels posteriorly, they are suitable for all levels of injury from the lumbosacral level up to the middle of the thoracic spine, and specially so for the usual sites of fracture in the lower half of the thoracic, and the upper half of the lumbar, spine. Velcro straps hold the corset together and there are no awkward buckles with which the arthritic fingers of the elderly have to deal.

FRACTURES OF THE PELVIS

Stable fractures of the pelvis are the rule and the same regime can be used as for fractures of the spine. The patient is assessed, carefully examined, radiographed and put to bed and sitting up is begun immediately. In a very short time the patient should be able to sit out of bed and again, once sitting, the pressures on the pelvis are not much different from those incurred by standing, particularly as most of the fractures occur in the ilio-pubic and ischio-pubic rami and rarely cause any disruption of the pelvic ring.

Very rarely an elderly patient does have a pelvic fracture which is unstable. A simple method of stabilising the pelvis by external fixation is to place two screws deeply into the ilium through the anterior superior iliac spines. The screws are then fixed to a turnbuckle crossbar which can be tightened so that the "open book" of the pelvis is drawn together anteriorly. With this apparatus the patient is immediately more mobile and may get up, sit, stand and walk. The fixation can be removed about three weeks after the injury (Figs 9 and 10).

FRACTURES OF THE RIBS

These are treated by activity, with a careful watch to ensure that respiration, being painful, is not so hampered that a broncho-pneumonia develops. This is likely to occur in the patient with chronic bronchitis because coughing causes severe pain and therefore is resisted by the patient.

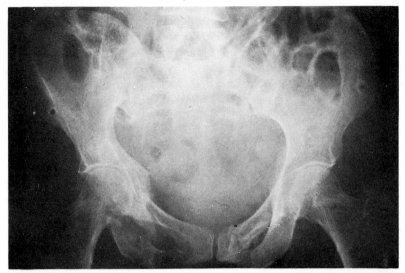

Fig. 9

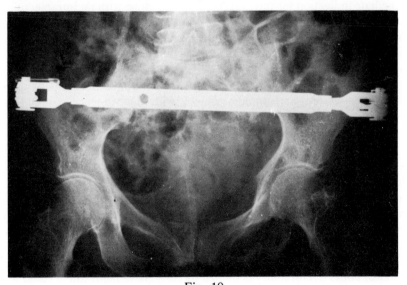

Fig. 10

FIGS. 9 and 10 The unstable fracture of the pelvis is rare in the elderly but this woman of 74 whose radiograph is shown in figure 9 was in great pain when she was admitted. Two days later she was treated by external fixation of the pelvis, using the "coathanger" technique (Fig. 10). The latter is merely two screws which can be fixed to a turnbuckle crossbar and then the tension can be increased to hold shut the "open book" of the pelvis. Note that the fracture runs down through the body of the right ilium, into the distal sacro-iliac joint, which is unusual, but that reduction after fixation was good.

Fractures of the Upper Limb

Fractures of the upper limb can be highly disabling either because of the pain that they cause or because they are bilateral. The active old lady with a bilateral Colles's fracture cannot maintain independence because she cannot manage all the activities of daily living, and particularly her toilet. Thus admission to hospital, or some other place of care, is necessary.

FRACTURES OF THE NECK OF THE HUMERUS

Most of these are impacted and require treatment, as an out-patient, with a collar and cuff sling. Early movements are started in the physiotherapy department for the first few days until the pain improves and then the patient is transferred for occupational therapy in the workshop where activities are graded to improve the range of movement of the shoulder.

Occasionally the fracture of the neck of the humerus is not impacted. It is then extremely painful. The patient is unable to maintain independence because any movement of the body produces pain. This situation is an immediate indication for internal fixation, best done with an intramedullary Rush pin. The technique is simple: through a small incision in the anterior fibres of the upper deltoid the head of the humerus is approached. A small hole is made for the introduction of the Rush pin which is then passed down and driven home moderately firmly with care not to cause the head of the humerus to split. This simple method so relieves the pain that the patient can start moving and may return home quickly with independence assured (Figs 11 to 13).

FRACTURES NEAR THE ELBOW

Most of the lesser fractures are separations of the olecranon process which should be treated by immediate internal fixation by whatever method is preferred, remembering that osteoporotic bone is not such good material as that found in the younger adult. Long screws, lag screws, wire, etc. may all be used according to the findings.

The old lady who falls on to the elbow has a special facility for producing "a bag of bones". This injury is treated by early movements and a collar and cuff sling. The pain, which may be severe at first, can be controlled by simple crepe bandaging which must not be too tight lest it obstruct the circulation. If this is still insufficient one plaster bandage to form an "eggshell" cast may be put on top of the crepe bandage but this must be taken off at about a week after the injury to allow the movements to start. Without early movements the elbow will become stiff and remain painful. Although full return of function to the elbow is very unlikely, the patient regains a useful arc of movement, with which she can manage all the necessary activities.

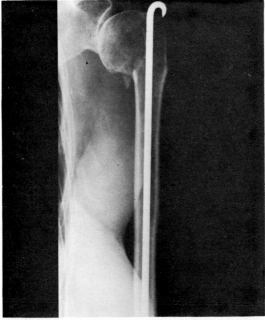

Fig. 11 The radiograph of a patient who had a very painful fracture of the surgical neck of the humerus. Simple pinning relieved the pain and the patient was then able to be independent with the use of a sling only.

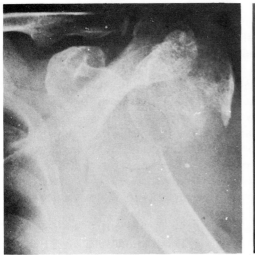

Fig. 12   Fig. 13

FIGS. 12 and 13 The radiographs of a severely displaced fracture of the neck of the humerus in a woman aged 89, who lived in an old people's home. The internal fixation was done "blind" through a small incision; the reduction was satisfactory, if not perfect; pain was relieved and mobility restored.

COLLES'S FRACTURE

This fracture, one of the commonest injuries of the elderly, should never cause disability and should not necessitate the patient having any interruption in home life unless it is bilateral.

The routine treatment is to manipulate as soon as possible under a general anaesthetic when the fracture is displaced and a plaster backslab is applied to below the elbow and bandaged in place. Immediate physiotherapy is given and the patient returns daily but has the plaster completed at the third day or later if swelling is still a problem. Once the plaster is completed the patient is then fit to attend regularly at the occupational therapy workshop where exercises are designed to preserve the muscle tone during the whole time that the plaster is on. It is not our practice to have further radiographs taken after the initial reduction if the latter was satisfactory; often there is return of some displacement but further manipulation will give much the same position though it may delay the return to function and give an end result that is less satisfactory than it would have been without the second interference (Pool, 1973). The old person accepts a less than perfect looking wrist provided it works well and without pain. If there is deformity at the end of treatment, it must be explained to the patient that it is acceptable because function has returned. Even at 80 an elderly patient will ask "Is arthritis likely to occur"? She must be reassured and she will then go home happily to use her wrist fully and freely.

Stress Fractures

Stress fractures are common in the geriatric population and osteoporosis, if it is accepted as a normal concomitant of old age, is certainly contributory to true stress fractures.

A stress fracture can be disabling if it is not recognised early. Similar fractures used to occur as the sequelae of radiotherapy but, with the improvement of technique, they have become rare.

In the geriatric patient there are many sites at which stress fractures occur and which can cause severe morbidity, or even death, from complications.

Any old person who has been on steroids must be doubly suspect for stress fractures because of the increase in osteoporosis caused by the drug. Such patients must be considered to be on the verge of having a stress fracture and they must be told to report any unusual ache or pain.

Stress fractures are often bilateral; should one hip have a stress fracture the opposite hip must be suspect. Fortunately it is rare for the stress fracture on both sides to develop at the same rate so that, as soon as one side has become slightly painful, there is a slowing up of activity and the less advanced stress fracture does not progress.

It is interesting to note that the stress fractures that occur in the elderly usually have a counterpart in children. Whether this is because the osteoporosis that may be present allows the bone to bend slightly more than in the ordinary adult or because of some other cause is not yet known.

SYMPTOMS OF STRESS FRACTURES

It is most important to recognise a stress fracture clinically because radiological confirmation often lags behind and valuable time may be lost.

Most stress fractures produce symptoms after exercise, mostly when it has been slightly unusual, such as extra walking, moving house, or, nowadays, being able to walk on a new hip or knee replacement to a greater extent than before operation.

The pain, of a dull aching nature, occurs at first after exercise but soon becomes continuous. There will have been no history of injury.

SIGNS OF A STRESS FRACTURE

There are only two signs of note; local tenderness at the site of the fracture and swelling, which, particularly if there is any other cause for oedema, may be considerable, especially in the foot and lower leg.

The important sites of stress fractures in the elderly are given below; but it is important to remember that practically any bone may sustain this condition (Devas, 1975).

THE PELVIS

Stress fractures of the ischio-pubic rami are common and in themselves are of no importance, but the pain that the condition causes is important. In the very old, it is a frightening, if not a severe, pain and it will put the patient off her feet until the condition is explained. The pain felt is in the region of the hip and groin and the symptoms, if not accompanied by a very careful examination, may be considered either to be coming from the lower abdomen or from the hip.

All four pubic rami may have stress fractures, but this is rare, and they do not necessarily all show at the same time.

Treatment is merely expectant and, under normal circumstances and with careful explanation of the cause of the pain, the patient does not need to be admitted to hospital.

STRESS FRACTURES OF THE NECK OF THE FEMUR

These can be very dangerous in the elderly. Some of them may occur as compression stress fractures (Devas, 1965) and are reasonably safe; if there is much pain then simple pinning of the fracture with one or more thin pins will be all that is needed to remove the pain from the patient and anxiety from the surgeon. However, a stress fracture which is visible, however small, in the upper surface of the femoral neck must always be treated as a surgical emergency (Figs 14 and 15), and the patient admitted at once for internal

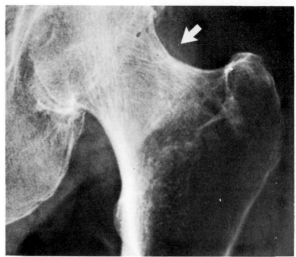

Fig. 14

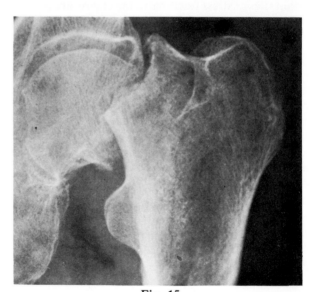

Fig. 15

FIGS. 14 and 15 A woman aged 56 had had long-standing osteoarthritis of the right
hip which caused her to take most of her weight on the left leg. Three weeks before
seeking advice she had considerable difficulty in standing with the weight on her left
leg and since then she had either rested in bed or in a chair. The first radiograph of
the left hip shows the beginning of a stress fracture in the superior surface of the neck
of the femur, which was not recognised as such. When she was seen again two months
later the fracture had become complete with considerable displacement (Fig. 15)
which necessitated a replacement prosthesis.

fixation. Often, however, the patient does not attend soon enough and the fracture becomes displaced.

It is not true that all fractured necks of femur in the very old are stress fractures but it is true that quite a lot are. When a patient is admitted to hospital with a fractured neck of femur with displacement, however carefully the history is taken, the patient may be in too much pain, too confused or too anxious to be able to give clear and coherent answers. Later, when the operation is over and the patient is hopefully looking forward to going home, careful questioning will often produce the answer that there had been some pain in the hip before the fall and that in falling the patient realised that there was a pain in the hip before she reached the floor. This history indicates that there had been a stress fracture which had become complete. The fracture may become complete either on its own, or by some trivial twist or jerk in the ordinary course of daily living. Once the stress fracture has become displaced it looks radiologically like any other fractured neck of femur and should be treated in the same way. It is in the diagnosis of the fracture before it has given way that the importance lies because this can prevent a considerable morbidity. If a stress fracture of the neck of the femur is diagnosed but there is no displacement, it should be treated by the insertion of one or more thin pins. There is one exception, and that is if the stress fracture is so very high as to be almost within the head of the femur. Then an immediate replacement is best because avascular necrosis of the femoral head is very common after this type of stress fracture (Figs 16 to 18).

THE TIBIA

One of the common stress fractures in old age is in the lower end of the tibia (Fig. 19) and quite often this is associated with a similar stress fracture at approximately the same level in the fibula. Less commonly the upper ends of the bones may be affected. Occasionally the old person will also develop a stress fracture in the centre shaft of the tibia and multiple stress fractures have been seen. Once the centre shaft has become affected by a stress fracture it is wisest to use internal fixation immediately because this means that the patient does not have to be in hospital for more than two or three days. The fixation need not be excessive. If the fracture is complete then an ordinary intramedullary nail should be used as described for fractures of the tibial shaft, but if it is merely very painful and still a partial stress fracture of the tibial shaft a thin pin passed down from the tibial plateau will be sufficient to control the excess stress and allow the bone to heal.

The stress fractures of the upper and lower ends of the tibia can be very slow to progress, very painful, very disabling and very difficult to treat. However, provided the patient is encouraged, and if the condition is explained to her, she will usually be able to be active, even if she has to be in sheltered care. She can still remain active, be up and walk to a certain extent each day. Under no circumstances should the patient be put to bed for "rest"

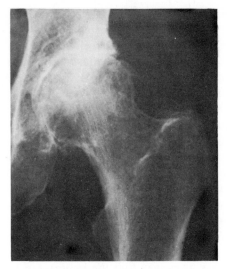

Fig. 16

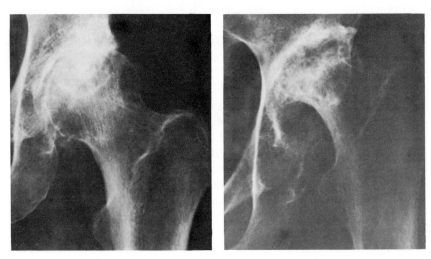

Fig. 17   Fig. 18

FIGS. 16 to 18 A woman of 76 had severe osteoarthritis of her left hip (Fig. 16). Five months later the radiograph (Fig. 17) showed increasing disorganisation, including the outline of the avascular part of the femoral head. The two radiographs when compared show that there has been a compression stress fracture running almost horizontally across the centre of the head of the femur with a slight alteration in the direction of the trabeculae. After a further three months disorganisation was complete (Fig. 18).

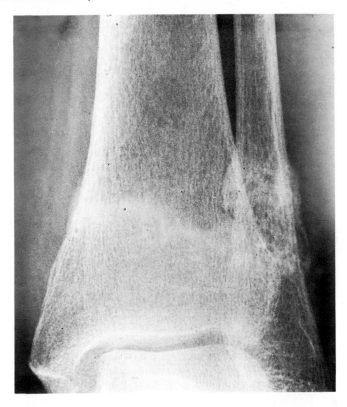

FIG. 19 A radiograph of the "common" simultaneous stress fracture of the tibia and fibula above the ankle in a 71 year old woman who had had pain and swelling for some two months. She said that she thought she must have strained it. She had noticed no bruising. She was otherwise well. She was given a supporting bandage and told to avoid walking so much that she got pain and with this regime she did very well.

and it should be in the last resort that a plaster cast is applied (Figs 20 to 23) and firm compression bandaging is by far the best treatment.

CALCANEUM

The elderly person does sustain that most interesting compression stress fracture of the calcaneum (Figs 24 and 25) and this can cause problems in diagnosis. However, provided it is remembered that it may take three months before there can be any radiological confirmation of this stress fracture and that the symptoms can be almost identical to those of the so-called plantar fasciitis, then, when the examination elicits tenderness on each side of the calcaneal tuberosity, the diagnosis can often be made. The patient may get better without any radiological confirmation. Treatment for this is reassurance, supportive bandaging, and a soft heel pad within the shoe. The

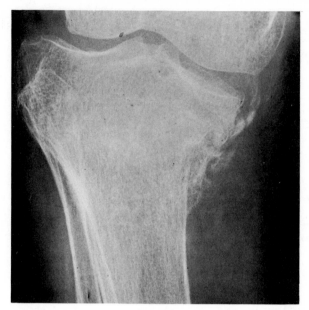

Fig. 20

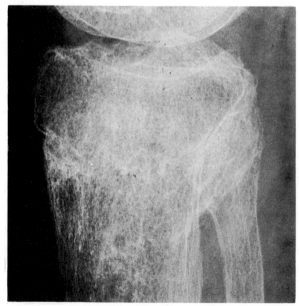

Fig. 21

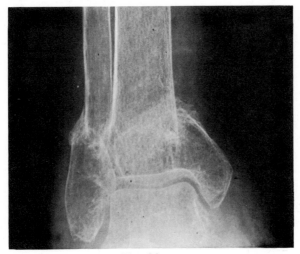

Fig. 22

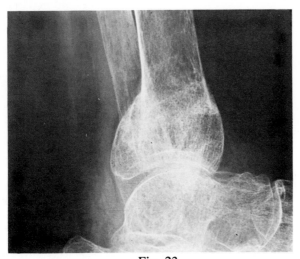

Fig. 23

FIGS. 20 to 23 A woman of 72 was thought to have a malabsorption syndrome and was being investigated for this as an in-patient when she developed pain in the leg. She had developed a stress fracture of the upper tibia (Figs. 20 and 21) and simultaneous stress fractures of the tibia and fibula at its lower end (Figs. 22 and 23).

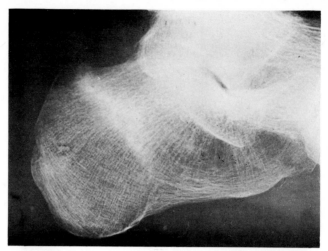

Fig. 24

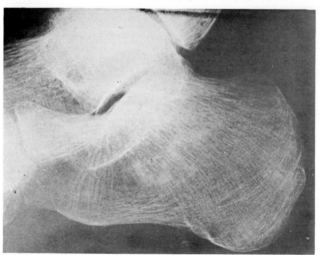

Fig. 25

FIGS. 24 and 25 A woman of 67 had had three weeks pain in the left heel. She also had had similar pain in the right heel five weeks previously, but it was less severe and it only lasted a week or two. The pain in the left heel got steadily worse each day, particularly after walking. She noticed that walking flat-footed caused less pain than walking properly. Swelling was always present around the heel at night but was better in the morning. Examination showed that both calcanii were extremely tender to pressure on their lateral aspects and in the centre of the tuberosity. Forced plantar flexion caused pain in the left heel. Apart from diabetes, the patient was otherwise healthy. A radiograph of the right, or painless, heel (Fig. 24) showed that there had been a stress fracture that was already disappearing, but the radiograph of the left heel (Fig. 25) showed a double stress fracture. Bilateral fractures of the calcaneum are common, as is a double fracture.

patient should be told to walk to the limit of getting pain. A high heel is also beneficial.

MARCH FRACTURES

Old people are subject to march fractures as much as the young person but here again a plaster cast is not necessary and usually elastic adhesive strapping, either alone or over some simple soft layer underneath, is sufficient.

The guiding rule in all stress fractures in the elderly is to continue activity as best possible without getting pain from the site of the fracture and to ensure that prophylactic fixation is done when necessary.

References

Devas, M. B. (1975). "Stress Fractures", Churchill Livingstone, Edinburgh.
Devas, M. B. (1965). Stress fractures of the femoral neck. *Journal of Bone and Joint Surgery* **47B,** No. 4.
Pool, C. J. F. (1973). Colles's fracture. A prospective study of treatment. *Journal of Bone and Joint Surgery* **55B,** No. 3.

11

Pathological Fractures

MICHAEL DEVAS

Introduction

A pathological fracture caused by malignant disease can be the final disaster to a patient of any age; it is particularly common in the older person. A bold orthopaedic approach will usually achieve not only success but the gratitude of the patient. However ill the patient is and however dire the general prognosis, no time should be lost in eliminating the fracture so that pain is relieved and mobility restored. Often this will allow the patient to return home where she may live out her remaining life independently and, perhaps, ultimately die there and not in hospital away from friends, relatives and her own personal surroundings. Often when the patient is presented to the surgeon she is ill and heavily sedated because of pain. Other bones and other systems may also be involved but, if there is a painful fracture present, or impending, it should be treated. There is no place for conservative treatment when an operation would relieve the pain and suffering. Never should it be considered that the spread of the cancer is so great that it is not worth operating. Even to restore the patient to a better quality of life for a week or two is sufficient indication to operate when an operation is possible. Like the very ill geriatric patient with a fracture near the hip, the fact that the prognosis is poor and that operation may have a very high mortality rate must not deter the surgeon from doing what is, after all, his prime duty, to ease the suffering of the patient (Figs 1 and 2).

Most old people are women and need to use a bedpan for micturition, but the surgeon, excluded by screens or curtains, rarely sees the suffering this entails; any form of lifting or moving a patient with a pathological fracture that has not been eliminated is painful.

For these reasons any patient with a pathological fracture from malignant disease must be considered as an emergency who will be best benefited by immediate operation. The haemoglobin content of such patients is low and blood must be given because, if an open reduction is to be done, the bleeding is often severe. After the operation, like many geriatric patients with ordinary fractures, the condition in general may be greatly improved.

From the point of view of the patient who has only a few weeks to live every hour is precious and, having been granted the knowledge that life is limited, the sensible old person accepts this with dignity but is anxious to make arrangements and to be as independent as possible during that time.

Some pathological fractures are caused by an obvious secondary deposit from a primary lesion which has been diagnosed and treated. Sometimes the pathological fracture is the first sign of the particular malignancy concerned. Some pathological fractures are caused by myelomatosis which is more common in the elderly than is generally supposed; these can be particularly difficult to diagnose because the radiological examination may reveal what appears to be an ordinary fracture from an injury and the underlying bone texture is not observed sufficiently keenly to recognise the slight changes present from the myelomatosis. If there is any doubt a bone biopsy taken at the time of the operation will settle the diagnosis satisfactorily. In any fracture in which a pathological cause is suspected a biopsy must be taken from the fracture site.

The other pathological fractures seen particularly in the elderly are those occurring secondary to the partial fractures seen in Paget's disease. Rarely these break spontaneously but often there is some trivial injury which completes one of the fractures. It is always necessary to assess the patient fully because to operate on a bone and secure one part with internal fixation after a fracture secondary to Paget's disease may allow the patient to break another fracture higher or lower which had not been included in the radiographic examination.

It is very important to have a full skeletal survey in all patients who have a pathological fracture to ensure that there is no other part at risk.

Pathological fractures that occur in the vertebrae are not necessarily obvious as fractures clinically; sometimes they cause only an exacerbation of backache, so that the possible consequence of paraparesis or paraplegia may not be considered and time is lost, thus giving a dismal prognosis which might have been prevented or improved by decompression; this is dealt with in Chapter 12.

Pathological Fractures from Metastatic Deposits

The bones most often involved and which can be satisfactorily treated surgically are the femur, the humerus and the tibia. It is the practice at Hastings to operate on all pathological fractures that are causing any form of loss of function in the elderly whenever this is possible. Fortunately those bones mentioned lend themselves very satisfactorily to internal fixation, provided this is done properly. There need be no hesitation in passing an intramedullary rod through a metastatic deposit. No fear of spread of the cancer down the nail or from fragments of the tumour being pushed down the medullary cavity should deter this treatment and experience has shown that the fear is unfounded.

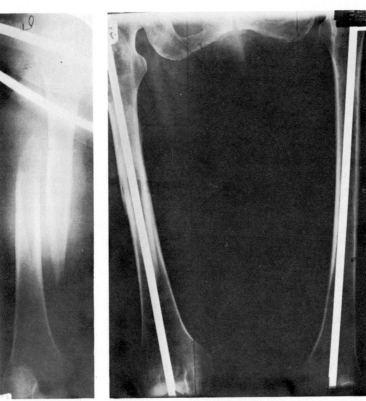

Fig. 1   Fig. 2

FIGS. 1 and 2 A very ill patient of 65 who had had a mastectomy for carcinoma of the breast had extensive secondary deposits in both femora with a pathological fracture on the right. She was in great pain. Both femora were treated by intramedullary fixation. The patient was extremely grateful for freedom from both pain and heavy sedation so that she could arrange her affairs, knowing she was dying, which she did eleven days later. Previously she had had a paraplegia from secondary deposits in the spine treated by decompression.

Most tumours that spread to bones are susceptible to one or another form of treatment by chemotherapy or radiotherapy, and the radiotherapist particularly is always grateful to have a pathological fracture securely fixed so that he is not hindered in the choosing of the ports of entry by plaster casts or other forms of splintage. Metal inside a bone under these circumstances is not a hindrance to radiotherapy nor need the fear that the metal will interfere with the treatment deter the radiologist.

When a patient is seen with a pathological fracture the previous history and condition should be investigated to make certain that the primary tumour is recognised; care must also be taken to make sure that the pathological fracture is not from a second primary lesion. If there is no obvious primary lesion and if a careful clinical examination supported by radiology does not indicate the site of the primary tumour there is the possibility of a "solitary" myeloma being the cause. It is not, however, necessary to delay operation for further investigations to determine the diagnosis because this will be most accurately done by examination of a biopsy specimen.

After the usual full clinical appreciation of the patient a skeletal survey must be done but with care so that it does not cause pain. It is quite sufficient to take two lateral views of the skull, one from each side, and antero-posterior views of the long bones and pelvis. The spine, if it is not clinically involved, will also be satisfactorily observed in antero-posterior views. Nevertheless it is most important to get good quality radiographs throughout and the lung fields and the thoracic cage are included. By this means any further lesion endangering the strength of a bone will then be seen so that special care will be taken of that part. Sometimes a second deposit may be so near to causing a pathological fracture that it is worth prophylactic strengthening of the bone before the fracture has occurred. For example, often if there are extensive secondaries in one femoral shaft which has a pathological fracture, a less advanced but similar situation may be present in the opposite femur; to introduce an intramedullary nail into both femora at the same time is simple and quick because the operation on the still intact femur will not need open reduction.

The clinical examination before operation may show spread of the tumour to other systems including the pleura and peritoneum with a consequent pleural effusion or ascites. This need not deter the surgeon from operating but the knowledge will be of value to the anaesthetist, who may aspirate the fluid from the pleura with a consequent, if temporary, improvement in ventilation.

A history from the relatives should be obtained, particularly if the patient has only recently been admitted to hospital; a change in behaviour or mental ability may indicate cerebral secondary deposits.

Sometimes, at a routine examination, a metastatic deposit is found in a long bone and the patient may be advised to have radiotherapy. Careful assessment of the strength of the bone is necessary because, after radiotherapy, the bone will continue to lose—or at the least not gain—strength for some six weeks; so if there is any doubt that a pathological fracture might occur then a prophylactic pinning or other operation should be done to ensure that a fracture does not occur.

If a secondary deposit, amenable to treatment, is found in a long bone the radiotherapist must be prepared to call for orthopaedic assistance if increasing pain at the site of the deposit, particularly on activity, indicates that the bone is at risk of a fracture.

There need be no fear about union of a pathological fracture. If the method of treatment is satisfactory union will normally occur but in those patients in whom the disease is so generalised or who are so enfeebled by their general condition that union is slow, the internal fixation properly done will be sufficient to control the fracture until death.

There also need be no fear that after an open reduction on a pathological fracture the tumour will fungate through the wound; this has never been our experience.

There is, therefore, no contra-indication to operating on a pathological fracture however ill the patient and however advanced the disease and even if it is only to make the patient more comfortable for a short while before death occurs.

SYMPTOMS AND SIGNS

Most pathological fractures are seen as an emergency which produces the immediate diagnosis, if not that of the underlying tumour. Before the fracture occurs it is possible to diagnose the condition and, forewarned, to prevent it.

There are two kinds of pain from metastatic deposits in bone. The first, which is certainly not always present, is a pain or ache which can only be ascribed to the malignant disease eroding bone or interfering with its blood supply, and especially the venous drainage. This pain can be very distressing even when there is no evidence of a fracture. The second kind of pain is that similar to a stress fracture; it is worse with use or activity and better with rest.

Any patient who attends with pain on activity or after activity and particularly if there is a history of a malignant tumour should be suspect. The symptoms of an impending pathological fracture are in many ways the same as those of a stress fracture because this is indeed what is happening.

The weakened bone is insufficiently strong to be able to maintain the stresses put upon it by the ordinary activities of living and thus at first there may be aching towards the evening or after activity, such as the morning shopping, but this ache will, at first, improve with rest at night or by day. The symptoms will gradually increase until pain is present all the time and it is at this stage that the unwary step will cause the bone to break completely. If these symptoms are recognised and a deposit is found in the bone concerned, then a full skeletal survey is done to eliminate other secondary deposits; because the curtailing of activity by pain in one leg, for example, may prevent another deposit, less advanced and in the opposite leg, from being sufficiently stressed to give rise to pain. If the symptoms are at all severe and if, radiologically, one cortex of the bone has been destroyed through more than a third of its circumference, then prophylactic nailing is necessary to stop a fracture occurring.

Very often patients with secondary deposits in bone are already bed or chair ridden by the primary disease, or by its spread to other organs, and it is important in such patients to pay great attention to any complaint of aching in the bones, whether in the limbs or at other sites, because the bone may break with simple nursing care. Unfortunately with bedrest many deposits may advance without symptoms and allow a fracture to occur with simple movement, the first complaint being of pain on movement at the fracture site.

Pathological Fractures near the Hip

The neck of the femur is commonly involved and the metastases causing the pathological fracture may also be in the head of the femur (Figs 3 and 4). The treatment is much the same as that for an ordinary fracture. The head and neck of the femur are resected and a replacement prosthesis inserted. There is no contra-indication to the use of cement. The important difference is that the rest of the shaft of the femur must be carefully assessed as far as the femoral condyles because if there are other deposits in the femur it may be necessary to use a long stemmed prosthesis which will pass down most of the femoral shaft; with this it is not necessary to use cement unless the upper part of the femur, at the level of the trochanters, is heavily involved and then the cement should only be in the upper part of the femoral shaft. This is because should further metastases develop in the femur below or at the bottom end of the stem of the prosthesis it is still possible to insert a Rush nail from below which will pass up the femoral shaft beside the lower end of the stem of the prosthesis. It is not necessary to delay operation to obtain specially prepared prostheses of the exact length required because although the ordinary intramedullary rod such as the Küntscher nail will not fit beside the stem of the prosthesis the thinner solid rods, such as the Rush nail, are adequate. They may be inserted from within the knee, through a hole in the intercondylar notch, as has been described for ordinary fractures of the femoral shaft in the elderly. Alternatively, solid nails can be inserted from the lateral aspect of either femoral condyles and this may be beneficial if one or other contains a deposit.

The patient should be allowed to walk the next day as usual.

Pathological Fractures near the Femoral Trochanters

Provided the femoral neck is not involved the ordinary technique of a pin and plate is adequate. As is usual, care must be taken to ensure that the plate obtains a sound grip on normal bone below the lesion or, if it is osteoporotic (which is often increased by the proximity of a metastatic deposit), a high density polythene plate should be used on the opposite side of the bone so that the screws will obtain a firm grip. Sometimes a longer plate has to be used. The care after operation is early mobilisation.

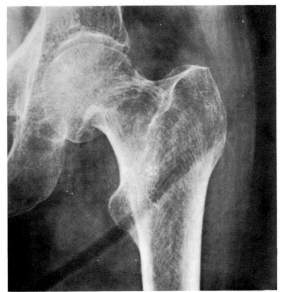

Fig. 3

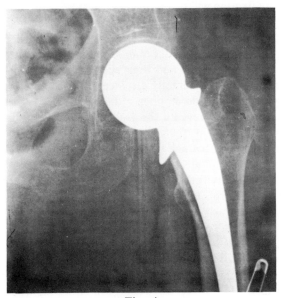

Fig. 4

FIGS. 3 and 4 A patient had pain in the hip for ten days, and the radiograph (Fig. 3) appeared to show a simple fracture of the femoral neck. On biopsy at operation a metastatic deposit was found. The hip was replaced in the usual way.

Pathological Fractures of the Femoral Shaft

It has been the experience at Hastings that a pathological fracture of the femoral shaft is best treated by fixation of the fracture with the largest intramedullary Küntscher nail that will pass up the shaft of the femur without it being reamed.

The technique of treating a fracture of the shaft of the femur in an elderly person by the insertion of an intramedullary rod through the knee has been described in Chapter 10 but, with pathological fractures, there are certain other points to be observed.

When a Küntscher nail or other intramedullary nail is inserted into the femoral shaft through a hole in the intercondylar notch, marrow and other tissue flows into the knee as the nail is pushed upwards. Although there has been no evidence that further tumour growth will occur in the knee, at the end of the operation the knee should be carefully washed out and the radiotherapist may wish to give the area of the knee some prophylactic radiation. It is unwise to ream the shaft of the femur which, already weakened by the deposit, may then split or break further. If, having inserted the nail, it does not seem to have a sufficiently firm grip, a second nail of sufficient length is stacked inside it, that is the two nails are interlocked, the second one passing up with one edge within the slot of the first nail. In this way a very satisfactory fixation will be obtained. It is more usual to have to do this for a fracture in the lowest third of the femur where the medulla is wider than above. Careful cementing of the hole in the intercondylar notch helps because it prevents further drainage of marrow and malignant tissue into the knee as well as preventing the nail from sliding downwards.

Even if the bone ends are greatly displaced it is usually possible to insert the nail without having to do an open reduction. This is because the usual loss of bone substance prevents the fracture from being impacted, thus preventing reduction, and also because pathological fractures do not normally occur with such violence that one end of the bone gets thrust through muscle, which can also prevent reduction.

The technique is to insert the guide wire upwards and, with simple traction and radiographic control, to advance it into the upper fragment. Normally this is done without much difficulty. The tumour around the fracture tends to shield the bone ends from gross displacement. However on those occasions when this is not possible, the small incision in the front of the thigh, sufficient to take one or two fingers, will enable the guide to be located in the upper fragment.

It is not necessary to use suction drainage in either the wound in the thigh or that in the knee after this procedure. Chemotherapy as a prophylactic is, however, useful because a patient debilitated by a malignant disease is more liable to become infected, even with commensal organisms.

Because the operation is done with the patient lying on the theatre table with both knees bent over the end, should the opposite femur also have a secondary deposit that causes the bone to be at risk of a fracture then prophylactic nailing should be done on that side. In the unbroken femur this takes only a few minutes. It will, particularly, relieve the pain that may have been present even at rest. This was done in the patient shown in Figures 1 and 2.

Pathological Fractures of the Femoral Condyles

When the tumour deposit is in one or both femoral condyles it may be very difficult to obtain a grip on the lower fragment without using some form of compression nail and plate.

Sometimes it is possible to pass a Rush nail through the lower part of one or both femoral condyles if there is still sufficient hard or healthy bone available to grip the hooked end; if this is done and firm fixation obtained the patient may well be able to bear weight without further protection. If this is not so, but having some fixation, a plaster cylinder is applied. This can be split for radiotherapy, or a removable plastic splint made. After the operation the pressure bandage round the knee can, if necessary, be coated with one or two plaster bandages to give an eggshell-like plaster which is quite sufficient immobilisation to allow the patient to be up and about until the proper plaster or plastic cylinder is applied.

Another method of treating the pathological fracture of the femoral condyles is to use the same method that has been described for ordinary supracondylar fractures of the femur, that is a compression nail plate. Polythene washers or a polythene plate on the opposite side to the metal plate are of value.

Pathological Fractures of the Tibia

These are rare because the secondary deposits often cause sufficient symptoms to make the patient seek advice before a fracture has occurred. If the patient is still walking and is found to have a metastatic deposit in the tibia it is best to do a prophylactic intramedullary nailing. This is done very simply by exposing the upper tibial plateau medial to the patellar ligament and, without having entered the synovial membrane of the knee, a hole is made in the front of the tibial plateau but as near the midline as possible and through this a suitable intramedullary nail can be passed down the tibial shaft (Figs 5 and 6). The operation is simple and quick and relieves the pain immediately and the patient can walk with safety while further treatment is being given.

Pathological Fractures of the Humerus

Although these do not prevent a patient walking often the fracture causes such pain that any movement is done with great unwillingness. Therefore it is necessary to fix the pathological fracture to relieve the pain. Even if there is no pain, and occasionally this is so, it is still important to fix the fracture because the difficulty of external immobilisation of the fracture is such that union will not occur; further, bulky splintage will seriously handicap the patient. Therefore fixation, by passing a sufficiently thick intramedullary

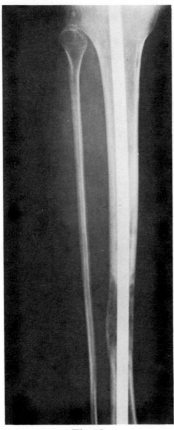

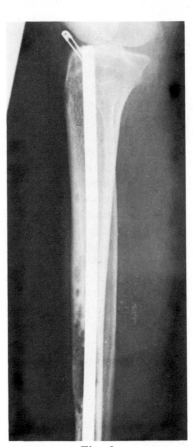

Fig. 5   Fig. 6

FIGS. 5 and 6 A patient of 72 had a simple mastectomy for carcinoma. One year later pain in one shin was diagnosed as caused by a secondary deposit and was treated by intramedullary nailing.

nail down the humeral shaft to the elbow, is necessary. The approach is from the outer aspect of the humeral head. This will not always completely prevent rotation of the fragments of bone one on the other but a collar and cuff sling is all that is necessary thereafter. Two thin nails may be used instead of one, and often this gives better control of rotation.

Other Pathological Fractures

Pathological fractures may occur in any bone in the body and, if they are of sufficient consequence to distress the patient so that independence is lost, any method of fixation available should be used to control the fracture and the pain. Any technique that may appear suitable to the occasion is justifiable, for even some control of the bones at the site of the fracture will add to the wellbeing of the patient, if only to give increased comfort and mobility in bed.

Myelomatosis

The main problem with myelomatosis in the elderly is not the obvious single myeloma that may be diagnosed before or after it has caused a pathological fracture, but multiple myelomatosis in which the lesion is widely spread in such a way that it is not necessarily obvious at the time when the patient first presents. Usually it is the femur near the hip that is affected and the very small discreet areas of translucency may not be recognised in the radiograph or may be considered part of the normal pattern of an aging and osteoporotic patient. The occasional history of pain preceding the fracture, particularly if it is in the femoral neck, may suggest that it was caused by stress; then the primary pathological process may go undetected for some considerable time. Myelomatosis must always be considered as a diagnosis in any form of fracture in the elderly which does not conform entirely to the normal pattern. It is far better to err on the side of taking a biopsy at the time of operation than to leave the question unsolved or, worse, unconsidered. The bone biopsy should be as large as possible because although the myelomatosis is diffuse it does not involve necessarily every fragment of bone.

Paget's Disease

The only problem in treating Paget's disease in the elderly is that some fractures are difficult technically because of the pre-existing deformity of the shaft of a bone or the occasional extreme hardness of the bone that can occur with this condition (Figs 7 and 8).

Provided proper fixation after reduction of a fracture through bone affected by Paget's disease is obtained, union will occur very readily. Often the problem is to obtain and maintain the reduction because normal methods of intramedullary nailing are not always feasible because of the deformity caused by the deforming aspect of the condition. Therefore it is important to use a technique which will take into account not only the fact that the bone is deformed but also that it may be very hard bone indeed; the unwary operator who sets out to insert a strong intramedullary nail into a shaft of femur with

Paget's disease may find that the nail gets jammed firmly in the cortex of the bone and will move neither forwards nor backwards.

Apart from technical difficulties which should not deter the experienced

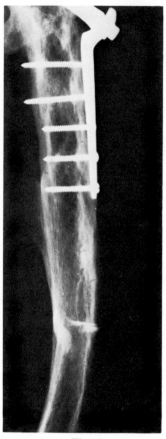

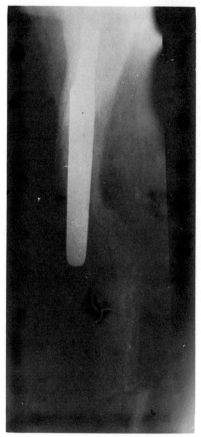

Fig. 7   Fig. 8

FIGS. 7 and 8 A patient aged 74 with Paget's disease. Notice how the fracture below the plate is hardly visible in the antero-posterior view, and how the deformity of the femoral shaft makes difficulty in fixation.

surgeon, all elderly people with Paget's disease should have their fractures treated in the normal way by immediate internal fixation.

Sarcoma secondary to Paget's disease is a well recognised condition but despite many old people with osteitis deformans in and around Hastings it has never been a serious problem numerically.

12

Paraplegia and Lumbar Stenosis

MICHAEL DEVAS

Introduction

Paraplegia is one of the greatest disasters that can afflict any person at any age. To the elderly it is usually the beginning of a terminal illness that immediately denies the patient independence of any sort whatsoever and is a condemnation to an ignominious and undignified death bed. The condition calls for the best resources of any orthopaedic unit that deals with geriatric patients.

Lumbar stenosis, on the other hand, is not so dramatic as paraplegia and does not deny the patient independence at home in the first instance. It is an insidious condition which causes weakness of the legs and a gradual disturbance of micturition leading to incontinence but so slowly that it is only gradually that the patient is unable to perform the activities of daily living; even this is masked if there is a relative or other help in the home. Only too often the whole syndrome is ascribed to old age. The essential lesion is a narrowing of the lumbar spinal canal, almost invariably from a degenerative condition. This may be a primary osteoarthritis or secondary to a previous injury or similar condition.

Paraplegia

In the elderly the usual cause is a malignant tumour involving the spinal cord, either directly or indirectly. Direct involvement is caused by the tumour tissue actually within the spinal canal and compressing the spinal cord; indirect involvement may be by the collapse of a vertebra in which there is a secondary deposit or even a myeloma.

It is important to have a prepared system of management for any geriatric patient admitted with a paraplegia because the speed with which it is treated will in great measure determine the prognosis. Perhaps the first point to be made is that it is entirely unimportant to try to diagnose the tumour. The emergency, and there is no greater emergency in geriatric orthopaedics, calls for the immediate relief of the pressure on the spinal cord at the earliest possible moment. Therefore any old person who is found to have a paraplegia or even a paraparesis should not be considered at leisure but must have an immediate myelograph (Fig. 1). This is because the myelograph will at once confirm whether or not there is pressure on the cord and the level at which it is situated. The usual investigations of the blood are done while the myelograph is under way, and at the same time the operation theatre is alerted. If there is a block to the column of dye then immediate decompression is necessary. Every hour lost reduces the possibility of a good prognosis and increases the chance of the patient lying paralysed and doubly incontinent for the few weeks of life remaining to them. Old people do not survive a paraplegia well.

PROCEDURE ON ADMISSION
The necessity for the myelograph is explained to the patient not only because it is an unpleasant and even frightening procedure, but also so that, if compression of the cord is not found, the patient will know why no operation can be done. A mild premedication, either an analgesic or a tranquilliser, is beneficial. Long and tiring clinical examinations to assess the level of the paraplegia from physical signs waste more time than they are worth.

Pain and tenderness are not very accurate as a means of locating the level of the lesion but careful palpation of the spine may give a rough indication of the site. There is one important pitfall in diagnosing the level of a paraplegia, and that is when a metastatic deposit involves more than one level or has invaded the canal and has spread up and down for a considerable distance.

Localisation by the level of the loss of sensibility is not reliable in early paraplegia. Previous radiographs may or may not have suggested the site of the lesion which is found anywhere from the high thoracic to the lumbo-sacral spine.

Myodil is instilled in the usual way and the opportunity taken to obtain cerebro-spinal fluid for examination and to note the pressure and its fluctuations.

If the patient is still able to sit it is preferable to use this position for the lumbar puncture. The patient sits on the edge of the bed, leaning forward supporting the arms on a table. The spine is cleansed in the usual way and local anaesthetic instilled. The lumbar puncture needle, instead of being inserted in the midline, is inserted about two centimetres laterally from the midline at the desired level, and pointed slightly upwards and medially to pass through the muscle, ligamentum flavum and the dura. This method is quick, easy, and carries much less discomfort than when the needle is inserted in the midline. If a "dry tap" is found, and persists after the usual manoeuvres, a different level is chosen. The pressure and colour of the fluid is

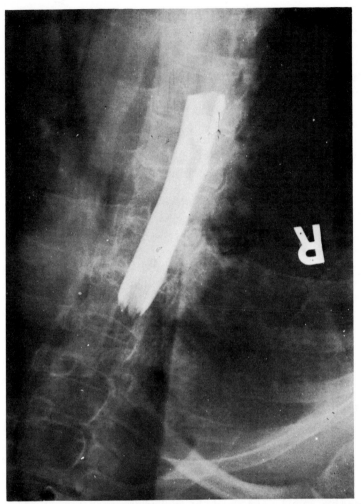

FIG. 1 A woman, seven years after a mastectomy, developed a paraplegia insidiously. When seen bladder paralysis was starting but was not complete. An immediate myelograph showed a complete block to the dye in the upper thoracic spine. The illustration is not upside down, but is in the same position as the patient on the tilting table, as is shown by the fluid level of the dye above. She obtained excellent recovery after decompression followed by removal of the adnexa and radiotherapy. The patient was lost to follow-up two years later when she emigrated.

noted and six to ten millilitres of cerebro-spinal fluid are withdrawn and the same quantity of Myodil instilled. The patient is maintained in a half sitting position while being taken to the radiology department.

The myelograph should be done in the presence of the surgeon who is going to operate. Sometimes if more than one area is compressed, some dye may trickle past the first block to show up a second. Also the level of compression may be seen to extend over several vertebrae and it is not easy to tell the exact level at which compression takes place. This tends to be found when there is direct involvement of the dura within the spinal canal, and especially with direct spread of tumours from the lung, and also with metastatic tumours from the breast or prostate. Should there be no block to the dye, then it is probable that arterial supply of the spinal cord has been damaged, and no surgical treatment will help.

DECOMPRESSION

The patient is prepared for the general anaesthetic and operation and as soon as possible taken to theatre for decompression of the spinal cord.

A long midline incision is made over the part of the spine involved and the spinous processes and interspinous ligaments removed as necessary until the lamina and ligamentum flavum are exposed. Often the tumour will have invaded the bone which may be very soft and occasionally almost pultaceous. A very careful surgical technique must be used to prevent damage to the underlying cord, which must be deroofed with great care, starting below the suspect area of compression and working upwards. When the actual area of compression is reached pulsation will be seen to return to the hitherto pulseless dura below that level.

It is not sufficient to leave the decompression thus, but the anterior surface of the cord must be explored to make sure that there has been no protrusion of bone from a compression fracture of a vertebral body, or that a disc has not been extruded, either of which may press on the cord and which may have precipitated the paraplegia. When the surgeon is satisfied that all pressure on the cord has been relieved, large pieces of gelatine foam are placed over the spinal cord. No attempt is made to graft the defect. The wound is closed without any form of internal fixation in the thoracic spine but if the deroofing has been sufficient to cause anxiety about instability for the lower thoracic spine from its eleventh vertebra downwards and for the lumbar spine, spinal plates should be applied. These should extend between healthy spinous processes above and below.

After operation the patient is returned to the ward and is allowed to lie flat to recover but intensive remedial therapy is started thereafter. It is often helpful to use an orthopaedic corset if the operation has been done in the lower spine but this is not essential. If there has been a complete bladder paralysis, regaining absolute control may take some while, but recovery should start within two or three days of the decompression: if it does not do so the prognosis is not good.

It is proper to operate on all patients with paraplegia from malignant disease even if the arrival at hospital has been delayed and if the outlook for recovery seems hopeless. This is for two different reasons. The first is that hope is given to all concerned, and especially to the patient. There can be nothing worse than to be afflicted with a paraplegia in the later stages of life and to feel that perhaps something could have been done but was not done. This also applies to the relatives and never will there be any recrimination on their part if the surgeon has explored and decompressed the spine but with no recovery of the lesion. It adds to the ability of the patient to withstand better her final illness knowing that all steps were taken that were possible.

The second advantage to operating is that it relieves pain and, from experiences of those patients who have lived for several months after a decompression, it does appear to benefit the skin, which is much easier to look after with a lessened risk of bedsores.

Lumbar Stenosis

Lumbar stenosis is the most bizarre condition that can deprive an old person of mobility. If walking is the most important physical sign in the elderly, then lumbar stenosis gradually reduces walking but in such a slow manner that the true diagnosis may be missed. It has not been seen other than in the lumbar spine.

It is one of the few conditions in the elderly that needs to have the diagnosis made entirely on the history and with no, or very few, clinical signs to go with it. Perhaps when there is a positive finding the most ominous is that of disturbance of micturition which may be either retention or a dribbling incontinence. This unfortunate presentation may well be seen by the urologist who, if he is not aware of the possibility of lumbar stenosis, may treat the condition ineffectually by local methods.

Never must the history be listened to more carefully than when an old person complains of a peculiar disability which may not even be referred to the legs. The history can take many forms. Characteristically one presenting sign is weakness of one or other leg, perhaps noticed when climbing a step or getting into a car and having difficulty when drawing up the second leg. Another presentation is a woolliness of feeling, a sense of unreality in walking, the desire not to go far, and the feeling that the legs do not belong to the patient. At other times there may be pain as a presenting symptom; pain in the back more often than pain of a sciatic distribution which is rare. However, if the backache is merely considered in itself the other bizarre symptoms which will still accompany the backache will not be discovered and simple measures only may be prescribed for the backache with the inevitable downhill progress of the patient.

Lumbar stenosis has many causes, from old injuries sustained in youth to nothing more substantial than some osteoarthritic lesions in the facet articulations (Figs 2 and 3). The spinal canal is essentially narrowed. This may be precipitated by a disc protruding; discs do protrude in the elderly and although they may occupy only a small extra space in the anterior part of the spinal canal this completes the stenosis.

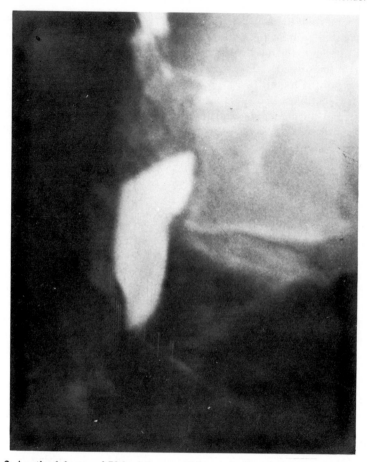

FIG. 2 A retired doctor of 70 had the most bizarre feelings in his legs and backache. He had had a fracture of the lumbar spine when he was blown up by a mine some 30 years before. The myelograph showed an almost complete block at the lumber three four level. The radiograph is upside down purposely in the position of the patient at that time.

No age is particularly prone to the condition but it appears to occur from late middle age onwards. One not uncommon cause is a spondylolisthesis from a degenerative arthritis so that the posterior and superior lip of the lower vertebra causes a compression of the spinal cord.

SYMPTOMS

As has been said above, these are most odd and great patience and tact is needed to get the whole story out of some old people who are inclined to be

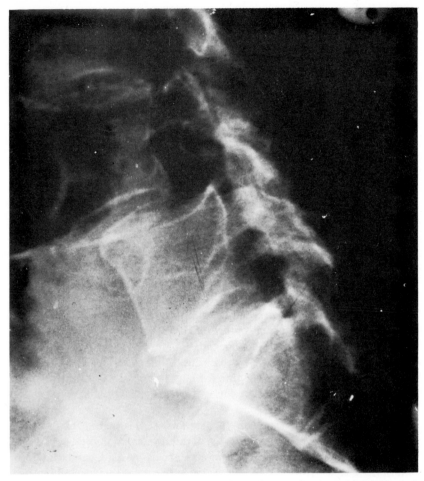

FIG. 3 Severe osteoarthritis of the lower lumbar spine causing a spondylolisthesis in a woman of 73, who could hardly walk. After decompression and fusion she was so improved that, six months later, she had a total hip replacement also for osteoarthritis.

embarrassed by the paucity of the more ominous symptoms that most patients feel must go with any complaint.

The patient will complain of going off her feet. This is the basic symptom but it may not have become complete, such as in the case of a person who only notices a little weakness in certain activities in one or both legs. Sometimes it is a relative or friend who says that the patient now sits all the time, whereas before she was a good walker and is now only able to totter from bed to chair to lavatory. Other patients may complain that whereas before they did their shopping and could walk there and back without trouble, they now find that every few yards they have to rest and, characteristically, to sit down or lean up against some support lest their legs give way completely. The fact that the normal history of bizarre symptoms may be reversed, that is the patient may find that lying and standing is better than sitting should not deter from considering the diagnosis. When it is appreciated that the lesion is caused by pressure on the spinal cord preventing an adequate blood supply, then it is readily accepted that various positions under various circumstances might improve or impede this blood supply. Normally the spinal canal is larger in the sitting position when the normal lumbar lordosis is decreased. Certain conditions may, however, reverse this and cause increased pressure in the sitting position.

With this in mind the further symptoms should be explored. Particular attention should be given to where the weakness appears to be, whether sensibility is altered either with pins and needles or numbness, whether feeling is disturbed in the feet, whether the balance is upset by lack of proprioception and, of course, great attention must be paid to any change in sphincter tone causing an alteration in micturition or defecation.

PHYSICAL SIGNS
A full, complete, careful examination will often reveal a healthy individual for her age with no abnormal clinical signs. The neurological picture in particular will be found to be normal. There will be no alteration of sensibility, all the reflexes will be present and there will be reasonably good muscle power and tone. At other times it may be found that there are some changes from the normal findings but these are usually slight and inconsistent.

It is important to try to establish the diagnosis clinically, but it can only be done definitively by myelography. As usual full investigation is done to ensure that there is no other cause for the lumbar stenosis than a local degenerative condition. A slow growing metastatic deposit from a distant tumour may have much the same presenting signs as may any other space occupying lesion and therefore it is important to exclude as best possible all other conditions by laboratory investigation.

Attempts at radiological assessment of the size of the spinal canal by measurements do not appear to be helpful; whatever the result, myelography should be done to determine accurately the site and length of the lesion.

TREATMENT
Occasionally a suitable support is helpful and should always be provided because even if it is insufficient it may well be necessary after operation. Physiotherapy is not helpful; the best treatment is decompression of the spine.

Myelography will have confirmed a stenosis. This may be partial or complete. Provided there is evidence of some compression and the history is typical in the sense that there is no other condition that will account for the weakness then laminectomy is indicated.

The procedure is essentially the same as that for paraplegia caused by secondary deposit but normally it is sufficient to decompress the posterior aspect of the spinal canal and to check that there is no great protrusion of a disc which has not been shown on the myelograph because the dye did not flow downwards or upwards past a complete block. The level of the stenosis is, however, usually below the third lumbar vertebra and therefore the myelograph should have been done by instilling the dye into a level above. Sometimes the plain radiograph will help in assessing the level of the stenosis.

A thorough decompression is necessary. If the lumbar spine thereafter appears stable no further treatment need be done. If it appears to be unstable and, taking into account the physique and general condition of the patient, it may be grafted. Gelatin sponge is first placed round the exposed dura; then a long strip of iliac bone is placed on each side with the periosteal surface deeply so that new bone does not grow and cause a further stenosis. Bone chips are placed on and around the long strips of iliac cortex, and held down with short cortical grafts lying crosswise. It is the practice at Hastings to hold the graft in place by the use of springs (Attenborough, 1975) which hold the cross pieces firmly against the rest of the graft. This has proved a highly satisfactory method because a dynamic compression of the graft is maintained and the spine is stabilised while the graft is uniting. This is because the springs are not rigid but give continuous compression, and some movement of the patient does not deter good union. The patients may, therefore, be mobilised rapidly. On those occasions when the laminectomy has been too extensive for grafting but the spine seems unstable, spinal plates are used.

The condition of lumbar stenosis is probably more common in elderly men than it is in elderly women. This is not to say that more men are seen with the condition but, because of the relative preponderance of females in the geriatric age groups, the fact that it has been seen in almost equal numbers in the sexes means that it occurs more often in men. There need be no hesitation in considering not only the diagnosis of lumbar stenosis in an old person but also, after careful enquiry into the activities of daily living and how the patient has altered over recent weeks or months, to take the decision to preserve a quality of life suitable to the patient by decompressing the spine at operation.

References

Attenborough, C. G. and Reynolds, M. T. (1975). Lumbo-sacral fusion with spring fixation. *Journal of Bone and Joint Surgery* **57B,** 283-288.

13

The Geriatric Amputee

MICHAEL DEVAS

The immediate and complete loss of independence caused by an amputation should not be a disaster to the geriatric patient provided the treatment follows the principles of geriatric orthopaedics of which the most important is to avoid decubitus and to restore independence. This is best achieved by the early walking of the patient.

The reasons for not leaving an old person in bed or in hospital for long have been gone into in Chapter 8 and this applies to the geriatric amputee. Most amputations in the elderly are done because of vascular disease, either simple arteriosclerosis or that precipitated by diabetes. Diabetes is common in the elderly, as has been seen in Chapter 5, and becomes more common as the patient gets older; any patient with vascular disease must be investigated very carefully for incipient diabetes.

No orthopaedic surgeon would consider an operation complete, for example when he had plated a fractured tibia, until he had put on the plaster cast and instructed the patient in walking with crutches, when to weightbear and when to have the plaster removed. There is also the fracture clinic at which the patient would be supervised. Yet the geriatric amputee does not normally get such service. Where amputations are closely supervised by vascular or orthopaedic surgeons and where there is an artificial limb centre close by ideal conditions exist, but most of the elderly people who suffer amputation are dealt with in small peripheral general hospitals far from centres and done by surgeons who may, perhaps, do three or four such amputations each year. This highlights the problem in one sense, that most amputations are not done by surgeons spending their time in doing amputations. To the vascular surgeon the amputation comes as a failure of vascular reconstruction and to the orthopaedic surgeon usually as a disaster he could better do without.

Hence it is not surprising that in the past there has not, perhaps, been the full interest that there should have been on the wellbeing of the amputee after the amputation has been done.

One factor militating against the geriatric amputee is that because most of the amputations are done for vascular disease and because vascular disease is almost invariably widespread there is often some mental impairment from arteriosclerosis and this may slow down the patient so that he is less vociferous about wishing to become independent and a form of apathy may spread over the patient and those who treat him.

Another factor is that many amputations have to be done as an emergency on a patient who is very ill with amputation as the last hope of saving the patient's life. The amputation having been done and the wound beginning to heal, the patient is often transferred to some other ward for further medical treatment so that the surgeon who did the amputation no longer sees the patient and assesses the day to day progress.

All these factors lead to poor after care of the geriatric amputee, particularly when it is shown that under ordinary circumstances the expectation of life thereafter is poor. Approximately one third of geriatric amputees die before two years are up and another third within four years. Many only survive for a few months but are never well enough to be able to leave hospital. Many will be too ill ever to be considered for an artificial leg and some will have already been chairbound or have had the opposite leg amputated previously.

Thus the quality of life in general that an elderly amputee can look forward to is dismal in the extreme. Half may achieve a satisfactory artificial limb and a third may survive for five years.

One of the problems about the proper treatment of a geriatric amputee is the inability of the patient to get to the artificial limb centre where the patient might be fitted with an early walking aid because many centres are far from the hospital in which the patient lies. Further, if the patient is ill she is unable to tolerate a journey from the hospital to the limb centre that may take up to two hours; and a similar journey back with a wait whilst she is measured or fitted of a varying, but often long, time. It is not surprising that many patients return exhausted, with many others too feeble to be sent to the limb fitting centre through no fault of anybody other than propinquity.

This was the experience at Hastings; the nearest limb fitting centre was very far away and it was found that the geriatric amputees were languishing in the ward untreated, unfit to go to the limb centre, confined to bed, or at best to be lifted out of bed into a chair for a short while each day with only the most fit being able to get up with some form of crutch or walking frame and hop a few steps. Even then it was found that the time taken to provide an artificial leg which was at that time of a standard and rather heavy variety suitable for lifelong use by a young adult, would often overtax such a patient's strength. It was, therefore, decided to introduce the early walking aid.

At its inception the early walking aid was designed as a simple support—a form of peg-leg—for the amputated side so that it would support the patient who might then walk using also a walking frame and achieve independence in the ward (Fig. 1).

The service was provided to the geriatric amputee who was too feeble, confused or ill to be sent to a limb fitting centre and who usually was being treated by the geriatric physician. The fate of these patients seemed far worse than that of the equally old, or even older, patient with the fractured neck of femur who was up and out of bed within a few days of admission to hospital (Devas, 1971).

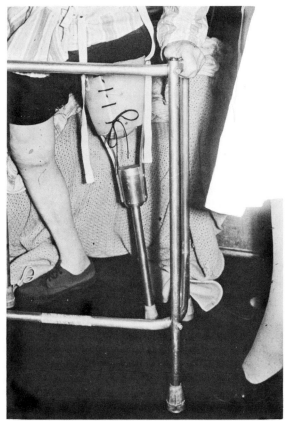

FIG. 1 The original early walking aid used at St. Helen's Hospital, Hastings.

The principle of early walking of geriatric amputees was simple. It was based on the fact that the old person should not lie in bed, that return to function was return to independence and that walking was the most important attribute of function in the elderly. It was felt that provided the patient could walk a short distance with a walking frame the quality of her life would be so greatly enhanced as to overcome any scruple about walking badly or deforming the stump. It was felt that any dangers inherent in the walking of these patients under such circumstances would be well compensated for by the better achievement of the amputees as a whole. It has already been said that the orthopaedic surgeon who denies an operation to his patient will preserve a lower mortality rate than he who operates freely on the elderly but that the latter will have the grateful patients. The same applies to the early walking of geriatric amputees (Devas, 1976).

A further benefit was found. The system was popular with the therapists who treated the patient because the effect of having and using an early walking aid raised not only the morale of the patient but of all those who treated her; the whole atmosphere changed from apathy and depression to one of hope and anticipation. The patient with her early walking aid beside her could look forward to walking, perhaps not today, but tomorrow if she felt like it. This boost to morale is so great that no patient should ever be denied an early walking aid however ill she is, because the mere sight of it encourages her to believe she will walk again. The fact that the patient does not wish to walk, or cannot walk, today does not mean that she will not walk tomorrow. There are, of course, exceptions to this. One example is the patient who comes into hospital in a wheelchair because of very severe heart failure, and will never be able to walk. It is obviously wrong to provide an early walking aid for such a patient.

The exercise of walking is good for the amputee and the development of the thigh muscles was better with an early walking aid than by trying to restore the muscle by physiotherapy; stump bandaging became less important because the exercise of walking restored muscle bulk and gave a satisfactory shape. Oedema was not a problem, also because of the muscle activity.

When the early walking aid was introduced most of the amputations were above knee, but with the years the level of the amputations became lower and with the long posterior flap the below knee amputation is achieving greater success than heretofore. Also over the years the early walking aid developed into a more sophisticated, but still simple, apparatus and is now manufactured on proper principles with a ready made socket that comes in various sizes; the simple side irons with knee hinges are easily adjusted and attached to the footpiece. The patient may have either an above knee or below knee early walking aid* (Figs 2 and 3).

It is very important that the early walking aid should be extremely light and it has been found best if it weighs no more than three to three and a half pounds (about 1.5 kilograms). The patient, relieved of the weight of one diseased limb, should not have the same weight replaced which will cause extra effort in walking. It was found that certain patients who had an early walking aid, when they transferred to a definitive limb of heavy construction immediately developed symptoms in the good remaining leg. It is particularly important now because of the preventive measures that are in use to prolong the life of the limb before amputation and no excess strain should be

---

*These early walking aids are made by Charles A. Blatchford & Sons Ltd., Lister Road, Basingstoke, Hants. RG22 4AH.

put on to the blood supply of the remaining limb even if this means a less sophisticated, but lighter, artificial leg.

The old person does not wish to work or walk long distances. There is no need for such a patient to be equipped with an artificial limb strong enough

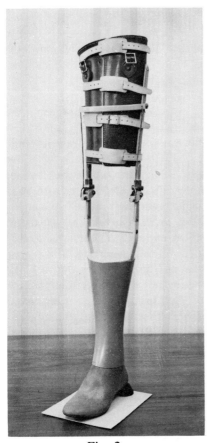 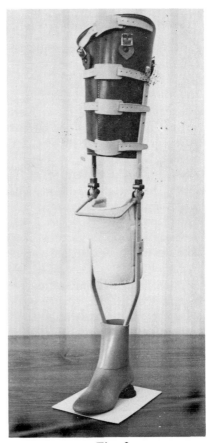

Fig. 2   Fig. 3

FIGS. 2 and 3 The enthusiasm of patients and staff for the original method of early rehabilitation ultimately evolved into the Blatchford Mark 1B early walking aid which is made for above knee (Fig. 2) and below knee (Fig. 3) amputees.

to last 30 years of active use and with a very high safety factor to accept the weight of the heaviest labourer. Instead the geriatric amputee would like a light artificial limb, easily put on, comfortable to wear and one which will allow independence around the house, the garden and down the street; it is very rare for a geriatric amputee to do more, and it is wrong that they should if arteriosclerosis is the cause of their amputation. Simpler and lighter artificial legs are now becoming available and with the advent of the below knee amputation it is often possible to do away with any support above the thigh. This is an immense improvement and one which has been found to be most helpful.

Prescription of the Early Walking Aid

It is the normal practice at Hastings that the surgeon who does the amputation should ask for the aid.

MEASUREMENT AND CONSTRUCTION

The measurements for the limb are taken by the therapist in charge and she will put them down on the form shown in Figure 4.

The orthopaedic technician fits together the parts and delivers it to the patient.

The early walking aid Mark II made by Blatchford comes with leather sockets lined with Plastazote. The separate side irons complete with knee hinges and locks are cut to length and bent to shape and fixed to a ready made footpiece which comes in varying sizes. A waist band is attached and the early walking aid is ready. It takes approximately two hours to assemble once the measurements have been obtained.

One of the advantages of using this form of construction is that a bulky dressing can be accommodated by bending the side irons directly so that the patient need not wait for the compression dressings to be taken off before starting to walk. Once the dressings have been removed the early walking aid can be readjusted to be more cosmetic in its appearance.

The patient is allowed to walk as soon as the surgeon concerned decrees. This system, which has been developed over 15 years, has been used with no obvious ill effects and no catastrophes.

If amputation is by election, then it is possible to measure the patient before amputation and have the early walking aid available at the earliest possible moment. This, in fact, used to be the practice and any amputee, except those who were admitted to hospital as an emergency and dealt with in the night, would be measured for the early walking aid which would be available when the patient awoke. However, experience showed that the average patient did not lose any ability to walk by resting for a few days after the amputation and before getting up but, on the other hand, fitting the aid to the patient and exercising the stump in bed with the aid attached was found to be beneficial. Many patients are too ill to be able to be assisted out of bed and it is important not to lose the confidence of the patient with the first few steps.

Cosmesis is important for two reasons, the first being for morale and the second that the slightly disorientated or fuddled patient will react far better to a cosmetic early walking aid, because at the bottom of the dressing gown

FORM OF REQUEST FOR AN EARLY WALKING AID (ST. HELEN'S HOSPITAL. HASTINGS)

REQUEST FOR EARLY WALKING AID

Hospital..Ward....................

Surname...Unit No..............

Christian names..............................Age...................

Address...

....

Date of operation....................

Diagnosis...

Date of request..

Surgeon...............................

---

1.   Left/Right leg   B/K   A/K   T/K

2.   Waist....................................

3.   Crotch to knee...........................

4.   Knee to heel............................

5.   Length of leg...........................

6.   Length of stump from crotch.............

7.   Length of stump from knee joint line.....

8.   Width of knee...........................

9.   Width of stump end......................

10. Circumference upper thigh................

11. Circumference middle thigh...............

12. Circumference lower thigh................

13. Waist to mid-thigh approx................

14. Shoe size...............................

FIG. 4 The simple measurements needed to make an early walking aid from "off the shelf" parts.

there will be a foot in a shoe: a rubber sheath over the lower end of the walking aid adds the semblance of a calf.

Many old people do have a reflex about walking in the same way that they have one about dressing. If they are fully dressed they should be up, if they are in a dressing gown they should be in bed. It is much easier to encourage a slightly demented geriatric patient to walk with two shoes on than it is with a pylon and a rocker. No patient need be considered too demented, too old or too frail for the prescription of an early walking aid; sometimes the prognosis may improve once some independence has been regained even if it is only around the ward.

Once the patient is safe on the aid, using a frame, and can walk alone, crutches or sticks may be tried. After the necessary wait for the wound to heal the patient can then go to the limb fitting centre to be measured for a definitive limb. Often various conditions will prevent this journey and the patient may have to exist on the early walking aid for many months. Under these circumstances it has been the policy at Hastings for the physiotherapist to maintain supervision and to ensure that the early walking aid is replaced should it show signs of wear or tear.

Some patients leave hospital with their early walking aids and never achieve a definitive limb. If their activity at home is limited by conditions other than the loss of the leg, it is better to leave them using the light and simple early walking aid with which to move around the house or across the road to the local inn rather than to subject them to the quite considerable rigours of having a definitive limb made.

Prevention of Amputation

In the geriatric patient with vascular disease great advances are now being made in the prevention of ischaemia using rhythmic pressure on part or the whole of the leg as necessary by air pulsation in an enclosed polythene bag which is wrapped round the leg. This is not necessarily the province of the orthopaedic surgeon but its use by vascular surgeons is increasing and it may well prevent, or delay, amputation. The fact that a patient with arteriosclerosis has had an amputation does not prolong the expectation of life; if the amputation can be prevented that expectation is not altered and the outlook for those who attend for prophylactic treatment will still be poor. This means that the limb may be preserved during the lifetime of the patient who is far better off with her own limb, which allows her to continue with independence without the necessity of an amputation and all the difficulties that may ensue.

The outlook for the geriatric amputee is not good; the Hastings experience is that 35% of geriatric amputees (in this context patients over the age of 50) are dead within six months of the amputation and that 50% are dead before two years are up. This means there is not much time left to the patient and no time must be wasted. Rehabilitating the geriatric amputee is a matter of great urgency and must be thorough and complete to allow the patient to go home to a quality of life that, if not of the best, is at least satisfactory because independence has been returned. Failure to practise such intensive methods, only made possible by a system of early walking, will often leave the patient wasting precious months of the few that remain sitting in a chair in a hospital ward to the detriment of all concerned.

References

Devas, M. B. (1971). Early walking of geriatric amputees. *British Medical Journal* 1, 394.
Devas, M. B. (1976). Surgery for the aged. *Annals of the Royal College of Surgeons of England* 58, 15-24.

14

The Geriatric Orthopaedic Unit

R. E. IRVINE and T. M. STROUTHIDIS

In old age a patient with a severe orthopaedic problem, such as a fracture near the hip, seldom has this as the only disability. In addition to the injury the patient is likely to have the same medical and social problems as those which are the daily concern of the geriatric physician. These difficulties frequently preclude early discharge from hospital and an orthopaedic department may find its beds blocked by elderly patients who have outstayed their need for purely surgical treatment. Eventually such patients may be referred to the geriatric department but by then valuable time has been lost. The patient's medical problems may not have been properly investigated or the social situation carefully assessed. Opportunities for rehabilitation and eventual resettlement may have been missed. This is all the more likely if, as happens at Hastings, the orthopaedic and geriatric departments are in two different hospitals several miles apart. In 1956 Dr L. H. Booth, who was then in charge of the geriatric department at St. Helen's Hospital, was quick to see the difficulties and offered the orthopaedic surgeons, based at the Royal East Sussex Hospital, some beds in a geriatric ward at St. Helen's Hospital, provided that they would maintain an interest in the patients transferred there and would visit them regularly. The collaboration which resulted proved so valuable that in 1962 a special ward was established for the assessment and rehabilitation of elderly women referred from the orthopaedic department. This was called the geriatric orthopaedic unit.

The Unit

The unit is separate from both the orthopaedic and the geriatric wards. It is run jointly by the geriatric physicians and the orthopaedic surgeons, who regard themselves not merely as responsible for each individual patient but also for the working of the unit as a whole. For administrative purposes the beds are separately classified as geriatric orthopaedic but the nursing staff qualify for the geriatric lead, an additional payment made to nurses who work in geriatric wards.

Operational Policy

The policy of the orthopaedic department is to operate on all patients with fractures near the hip as early as possible. Apart from life-threatening heart failure and unstable diabetes, medical complications are better investigated and treated once the fracture has been dealt with. Afterwards, to separate the ill geriatric patients from the main stream of the orthopaedic ward allows their concurrent illnesses to be investigated and treated and their rehabilitation to proceed in an atmosphere appropriate to their needs. To have such geriatric orthopaedic patients in one ward makes it easier to coordinate the efforts of all the members of the team and prevents argument about which patients should be transferred and when. Selection of patients for the orthopaedic geriatric unit is in the hands of the orthopaedic surgeons. Most patients do well in the orthopaedic ward alone but about one third need the special facilities of the unit. The unit is not a convalescent ward and the patients who are most ill and therefore most in need of medical treatment are given priority.

Transfer to the geriatric orthopaedic unit involves the patients in a move from one ward to another and in Hastings from one hospital to another. This may be alarming and sometimes confusing to the patient. Special efforts are made by the staff to combat this by a friendly welcome on arrival. A booklet with information about the hospital is provided and the name of the patient is written in large letters on a card attached to the bedside locker so that all the staff may immediately identify her.

The patient is, of course, accompanied by the medical and nursing notes but the sister of the geriatric orthopaedic unit has to re-assess the nursing needs. Nursing care is offered in one of four grades and an appropriate coloured symbol is placed by the patient's bed. A blue star indicates that she has a pressure sore or is at risk for one and must be turned two hourly when in bed and encouraged to move in the chair every two hours when she is up. A yellow star indicates that she is not at risk for pressure sores but is not yet well enough for strenuous rehabilitation. A green star indicates that she should be encouraged to make every effort to help herself and in particular should walk to the lavatory with as much assistance as she requires. A red star indicates that she is capable of self care and should not need any assistance.

Aims of the Unit

The unit offers the patient the same sort of assessment as is given to all other patients admitted to the geriatric unit. This involves consideration of the physical, psychological, functional and social problems of the patient and aims to restore her to the greatest possible degree of independence. The combined clinical approach and joint planning of the rehabilitation programme creates an atmosphere of co-operation between the two departments. It ensures that the acute orthopaedic wards are not required to provide prolonged care for patients whose needs are no longer surgical and it ensures that the geriatric department receives prompt orthopaedic treatment for those patients who require it.

The Ward

The ward must have equipment suitable for geriatric rehabilitation. The most important tools for this purpose are the bed, the wardrobe locker, the chair and the table (Figs 1 to 4). The bed must be of adjustable height. The patient must be able to sit on it with her feet touching the floor so that she can get in and out without being lifted. At the same time it is convenient for the nurse to be able to raise the bed should the patient become ill enough to require bedside nursing. It is also helpful to the nurse to be able to make the bed without straining her back. If necessary, before the patient is discharged, the patient can have the bed adjusted to the height of her own bed at home. The best adjustable height beds are the pedal operated models made to the Kings Fund design. It is also necessary to have one or two water beds for patients with pressure sores (see chapter 2).

CHAIRS
The ward must have a variety of chairs since no one design can suit everybody. In general an old person's chair should have a fairly high seat, about 450 millimetres (18 inches) from the floor. The arms should come well forward to give support when standing up and sitting down. A high back is an advantage with a bulge to support the lumbar lordosis. Wings are popular because they exclude draughts. Many geriatric chairs incorporate a foot rest which must be folded or slid out of the way when the patient stands up. Most chairs are now made with small wheels to facilitate movement, but it is vital that they should be braked when the chair is stationary. Some patients feel more secure in a chair with a detachable tray. Others resent trays and feel imprisoned. Trays should never be used to restrain a restless patient. The most useful general purpose chairs for a geriatric ward are the McLaughlin Offerton chair and the Ness Tyne chair. A chair of adjustable height such as the Doherty Easy to Rise model is convenient for assessment.

A tilting chair is popular with some feeble patients when they want to take a nap. It is also very useful for patients with postural hypotension who feel faint when they sit upright. A suitable tilting chair is the McLaughlin Buxton model.

An ejector or self lift chair is helpful to some patients in the early stages of rehabilitation. The seat springs upward as the patient leans forward, helping her to her feet. The Bromsgrove model is suitable.

Every ward should have a wheelchair and a sanitary chair is of value provided it is not used for patients who should be walking to the lavatory.

LOCKER

It is most important that the patient should be dressed each day. The St. Helen's wardrobe locker provides a convenient means of keeping the

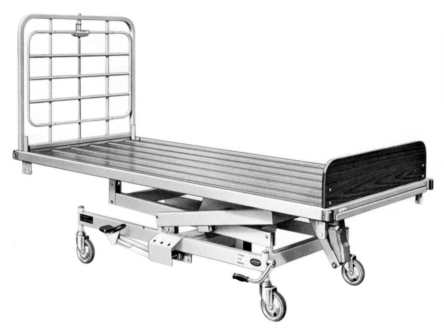

FIG. 1 An adjustable height bed (Kings Fund design) which is easy to operate both in altering the height or in moving the bed.

patient's clothes and personal belongings by her bed. A ward needs some left hand as well as right hand lockers. Patients are expected not only to dress but to wear shoes rather than bedroom slippers, as these make walking easier and safer. Remploy felt boots are useful for patients with deformed or swollen feet. It is most important that the patient should be up and dressed for the weekly ward round which, psychologically, is the most important event in her week and shows her that she is on the way home. To confiscate a patient's clothes and leave her in a nightdress, dressing gown and slippers makes her feel an invalid and lowers her self esteem. It also deprives her of some useful physiotherapy because the act of dressing exercises every joint in the body.

DAY SPACE

If possible the ward should have a day room and a dining area. It is a great help to the patient's morale to sit at a table. To walk to a meal even if the dining area is only a few feet away, exercises the limbs and advances the patient's rehabilitation. Lavatories, as in every geriatric ward, should be near at hand. The problem of incontinence is greatly reduced in a favourable environment with easy access to the toilet. All patients in a geriatric ward,

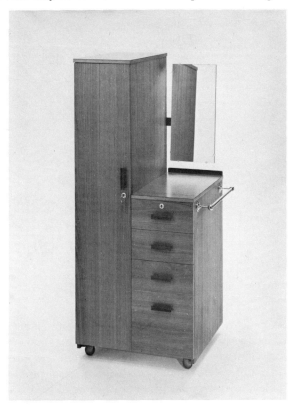

FIG. 2 The St. Helen's locker is made in left and right hand units. It offers some privacy between patients but, most important, holds the clothes of the patient who may then learn to dress herself each day.

whether in bed or in a day room, should be within 10 metres of a lavatory. Lavatories should be fitted with suitable rails. At least one should have a raised seat. Another should be wide enough to take a wheelchair.

It is a great advantage if the patient can have a commode at her bedside at night. If every patient has her own bedside commode the bedpan becomes virtually obsolete. The Zimmer Mayfair commode with a detachable receptacle can conveniently double as a bedside commode or sanitary chair. When it is used as a static commode the wheels must be braked.

Method of Assessment

The day to day care is provided by the junior staff of the geriatric unit. One of the two pre-registration house physicians in the geriatric unit has the orthopaedic geriatric ward as part of his responsibility. He is supervised by the senior house officer, the registrar and the senior registrar. In taking the history particular attention is paid to the circumstances which led to the

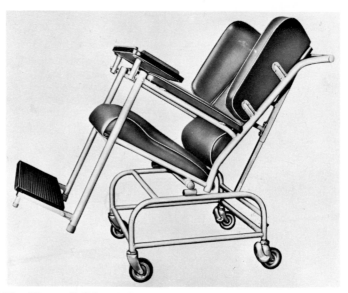

FIG. 3 The "Buxton" tilting chair (McLoughlin) which is very useful for the patient with postural hypotension.

injury in order to define the reason for the fall. Careful clinical examination follows including an assessment of the patient's mental and emotional state.

In the elderly multiple pathology is the rule and complete assessment should lead to a full understanding of all the medical problems. We have found the problem orientated medical record to be of great value and when the house physician goes round with the registrar or senior registrar a medical problem list is written. The physiotherapist, the occupational therapist and social worker make their own assessment of the patient as soon as possible after transfer.

The patient would be justifiably bewildered if each member of the team took decisions about his future without consulting the others. It is therefore essential for all to meet weekly on the ward round and discuss with the patient the plans for her rehabilitation.

COMBINED ROUND

The central event of the week is therefore the combined round, conducted by the orthopaedic surgeon and geriatric physician. The round is attended also by members of the junior medical staff of the orthopaedic and geriatric departments, by the nursing staff, the physiotherapists, the occupational therapists and the medical social worker. All problems, medical, surgical, social and functional can then be considered. A complete assessment is made and any problems which have to be dealt with by any member of the team can be decided immediately. Communication is thus achieved with speed and

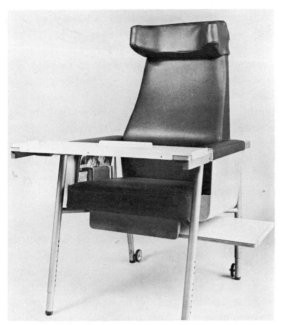

FIG. 4 The "Easy to rise" chair (Doherty) greatly encourages independence in the ward.

understanding. This increases the tempo of rehabilitation and ensures a more efficient use of hospital beds.

During the ward round and in all daily routine the patient must be fully involved. Often slight deafness or mental infirmity makes it hard for her to participate in the discussion. If she does not understand what is going on she may become frightened, confused or unwilling to try. It is distressing for any old person to be separated from home. She needs assurance not only that she will go home in due time but also that she will not be asked to go until she is ready.

At the same time the presence of such a large team of experts may in itself be alarming. All members of the team realise that it may be better to go back and have a quiet word with her about some specific difficulty when the round is over.

The relatives must also be kept in the picture. The ward should have open visiting and relatives should be welcome at any time. Consultants should be willing to discuss with them the problems of the patient's progress and future care.

Rehabilitation Programme

Progress in rehabilitation can only be expected when the patient's medical and surgical problems have been properly attended to. Physiotherapy is carried out mainly on the ward because in this way the staff become aware of the patient's progress and the treatment loses its mystique. What produces results is perseverance and frequent attempts at walking. Training by the physiotherapist should be supplemented by practice supervised by physiotherapy helpers.

The first attempts at walking are often best made between parallel bars which help to restore confidence. The best walking aid for the elderly geriatric orthopaedic patient is usually a walking frame, but if she is very unsteady a Rollator, a frame with wheels providing some resistance to tipping backwards, is very useful. Having learned to walk on the level, the patient should practise on stairs. Her performance in the lavatory should also be assessed. Once she has regained her confidence, the physiotherapist will teach her how to pick herself up should she fall again.

The occupational therapist assesses the patient as soon as possible and assists her in the activities of daily living. Equipped with information provided by the social worker about the patient's home circumstances, she can then plan a programme of activity. Emphasis in occupational therapy should be on dressing, cooking and self help activities generally. It is a great advantage if the patient can go from the ward to the occupational therapy department or day hospital with its kitchen, assessment room, assisted bathroom and facilities for recreation.

The nurse in the orthopaedic geriatric unit has the most difficult role of any member of the team. She has to provide tender loving care to a patient who has been through a frightening experience. She gives the medicines, dresses the wound and may need to pay attention to pressure sores. In addition however, she must see herself as the person who extends the patient's rehabilitation programme. No professional therapist, even with a helper, can offer the patient more than a short period of treatment each day. What is gained from this depends upon the help and encouragement offered at other times, particularly by the nurse. In rehabilitation the central activity of the nurse is to help the patient with dressing and to assist her to walk to the lavatory.

Rehabilitation must not become a fetish and in a situation where at least a quarter of the patients are going to die it is important that the staff recognise when the patient is dying and when further attempts at enthusiastic medical treatment and rehabilitation become fruitless and inhumane. The nurse is often a better judge of this situation than is the doctor, particularly if he is relatively junior. The nurse should never hesitate to make her views known to the doctor because her intimate contact with the patient often gives her the best picture of the whole situation.

The social worker provides a crucial contribution to the work of the team. She helps the patient to come to terms with what has happened to her. She helps her to cope with the bewildering demands and expectations of other members of the team. It is her concern to find out about the home circumstances and about the needs and feelings of the relatives. These she interprets to other members of the team and her contribution plays a vital role in determining the rehabilitation programme. If the patient cannot return to her previous environment it is the social worker's responsibility to find alternative accommodation more suited to her needs.

Outcome

The patient remains in the geriatric orthopaedic unit for some three to five weeks. Once it is clear that her continuing need for hospital treatment is no longer determined by the orthopaedic lesion but by her general medical condition, the patient becomes the sole responsibility of the geriatric department and is transferred to one of its general wards for continuing care.

In practice about two thirds of the patients are able to be discharged. Most of those who come from their own homes are able to return there but some patients, after the fracture, require more care and support than is available to them at home. They need residential care. Of those admitted from their own homes about 20% die. People who are already so frail that they need care in an old people's home before the fracture have a much higher mortality, over 50%. For a few patients whose needs cannot be met in any other way the geriatric unit undertakes to provide continuing care. Three-quarters of those who die do so in the first six weeks after admission to hospital.

Conclusion

The orthopaedic geriatric unit at Hastings has now been running for more than 15 years. It has provided a welcome forum for collaboration between the orthopaedic and geriatric departments and has promoted co-operative attitudes on both sides. Because a ward is clearly earmarked for this purpose the geriatric department does not feel that the orthopaedic patients are in competition with the many other calls upon its facilities. The fact that the orthopaedic department treats the whole exercise as one of genuine consultation and not simply as a convenient way to offload its failures upon a clinical undertaker has set a pattern of co-operation which makes the whole exercise a pleasure and greatly benefits the patient.

Further Reading

Clark, A. N. G. and Wainwright, D. (1966). The management of the fractured neck of femur in the elderly female. A joint approach of orthopaedic surgery and geriatric medicine. *Gerontologica Clinica* **8,** 321-326.

Devas, M. B. (1964). Fractures in the elderly. *Gerontologica Clinica* **6,** 347-359.

Devas, M. B. (1970). The treatment of patients with fractures near the hip. *Modern Geriatrics* **1,** 45-53.

Devas, M. B. (1974). Geriatric orthopaedics. *British Medical Journal* **1,** 190-192.

Devas, M. B. and Irvine, R. E. (1963). The geriatric orthopaedic unit. *Journal of Bone and Joint Surgery* **46B,** 630.

Devas, M. B. and Irvine, R. E. (1969). The geriatric orthopaedic unit. *British Journal of Geriatric Practice* **6,** 19-25.

Devas, M. B. and Marr, J. D. (1968). A geriatric orthopaedic unit. *Nursing Mirror* **126,** 25.

Irvine, R. E. and Devas, M. B. (1964). "Fractured neck of femur in elderly women. Age with a Future". p. 276. Munksgaard, Copenhagen.

Irvine, R. E., Bagnall, M. K. and Smith, B. J. (1977). "The Older Patient", 3rd Edn. English Universities Press, London.

McIntyre, N. (1973). The problem orientated medical record. *British Medical Journal* **2,** 598-600.

Thomas, T. G. and Stevens, R. S. (1974). Social effects of fractures of the neck of the femur. *British Medical Journal* **3,** 456-458.

Index